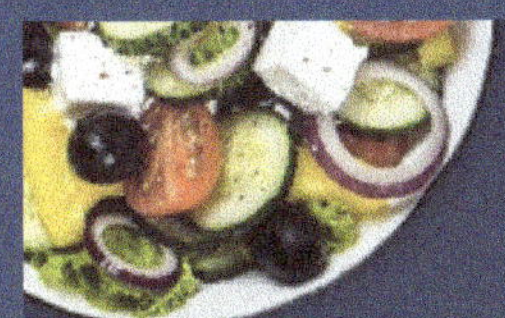

2024

MEDITERRANEAN
DIET COOKBOOK FOR TWO

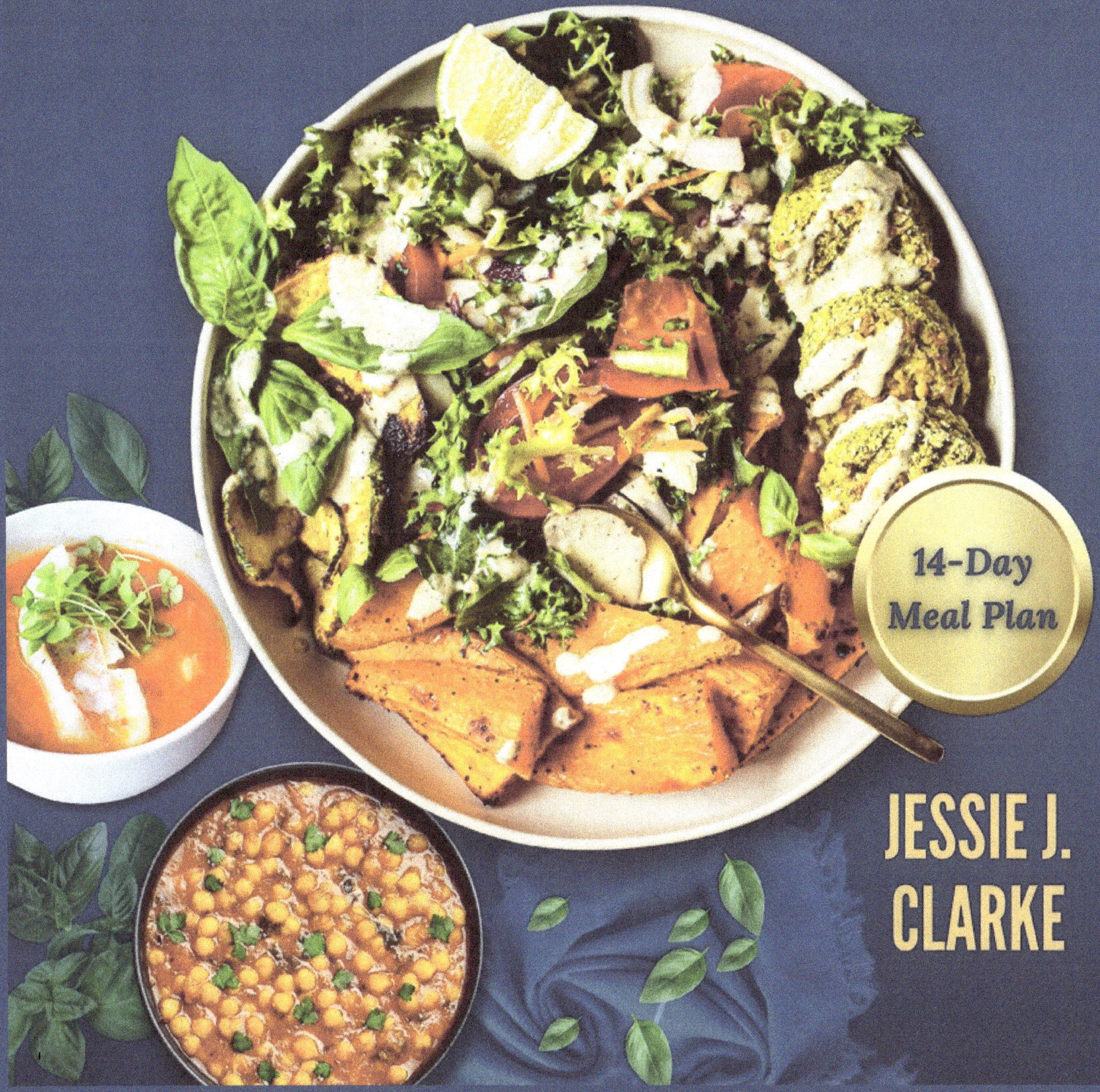

14-Day
Meal Plan

JESSIE J. CLARKE

MEDITERRANEAN DIET COOKBOOK FOR TWO 2024

The Complete Beginner's Guide to Perfect Wellness With Over 50+ Simple and Delicious Recipes for Healthy Eating, And Culinary Bliss

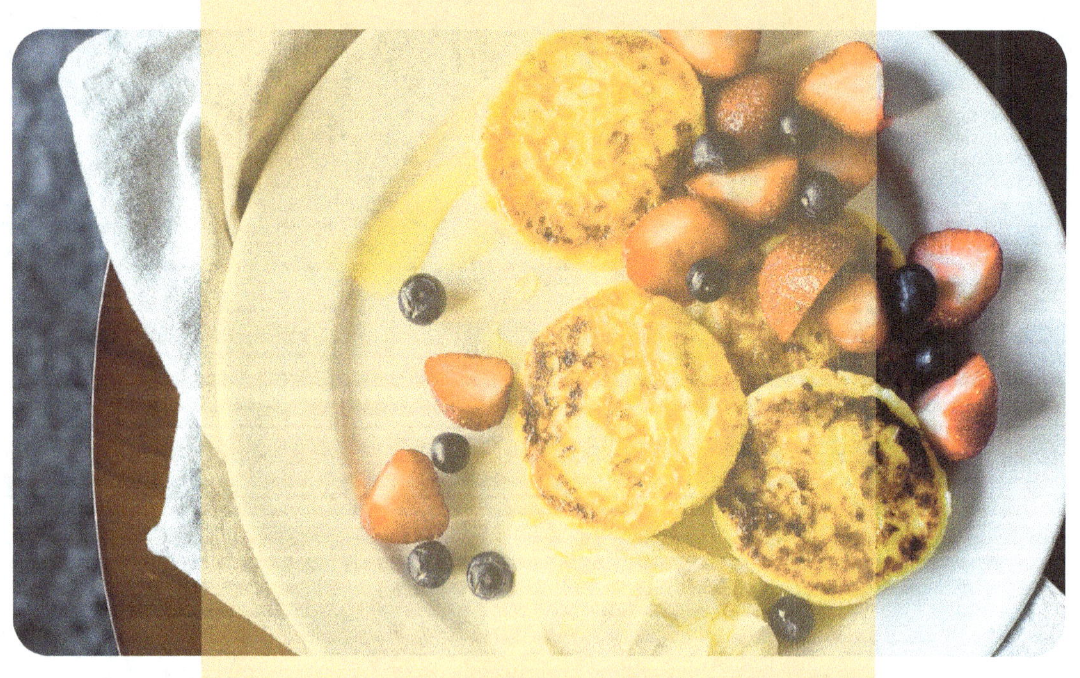

JESSIE J. CLARKE

TABLE OF CONTENTS

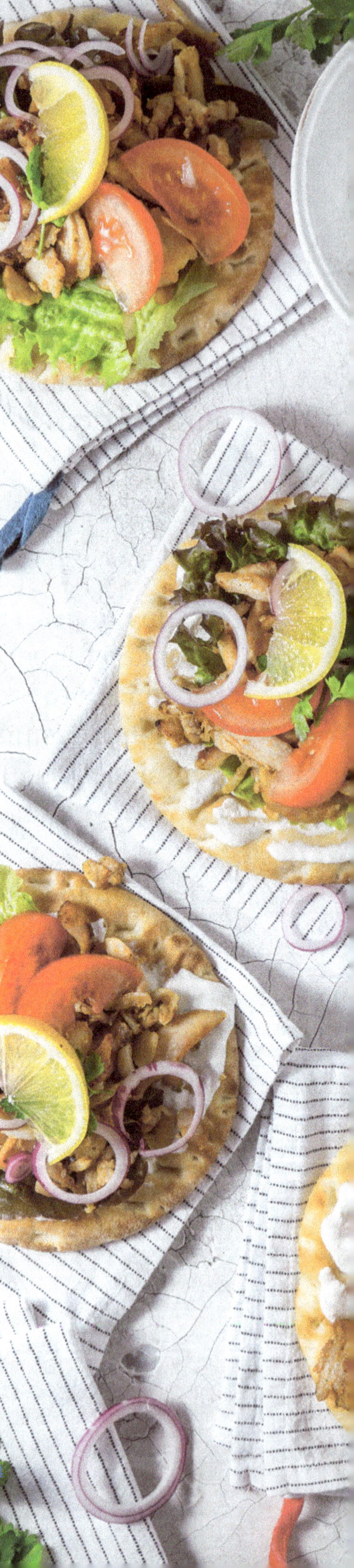

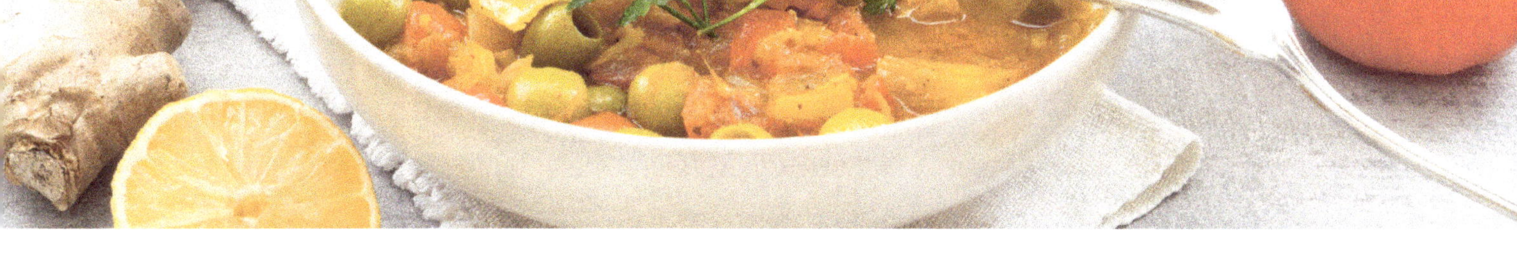

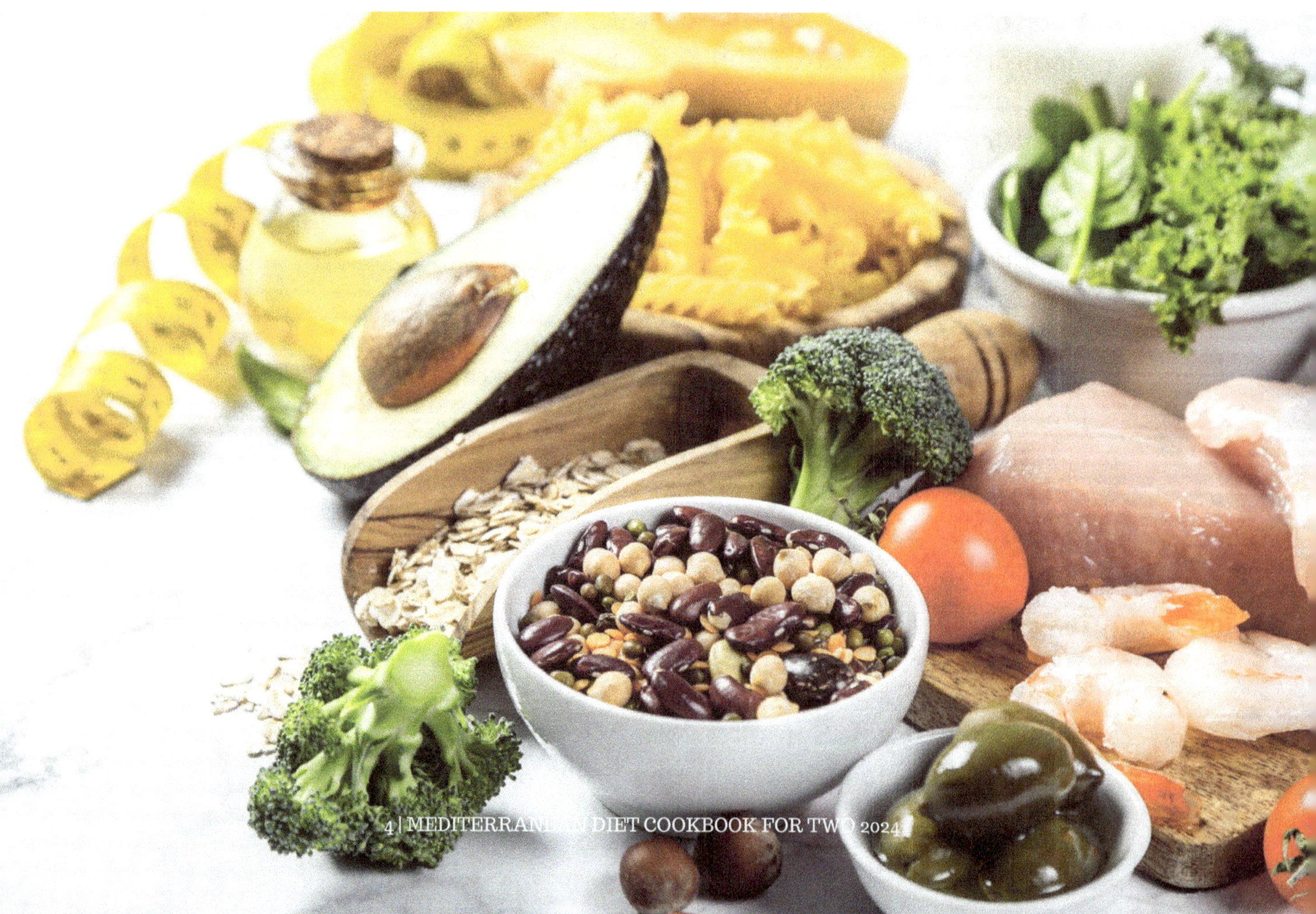

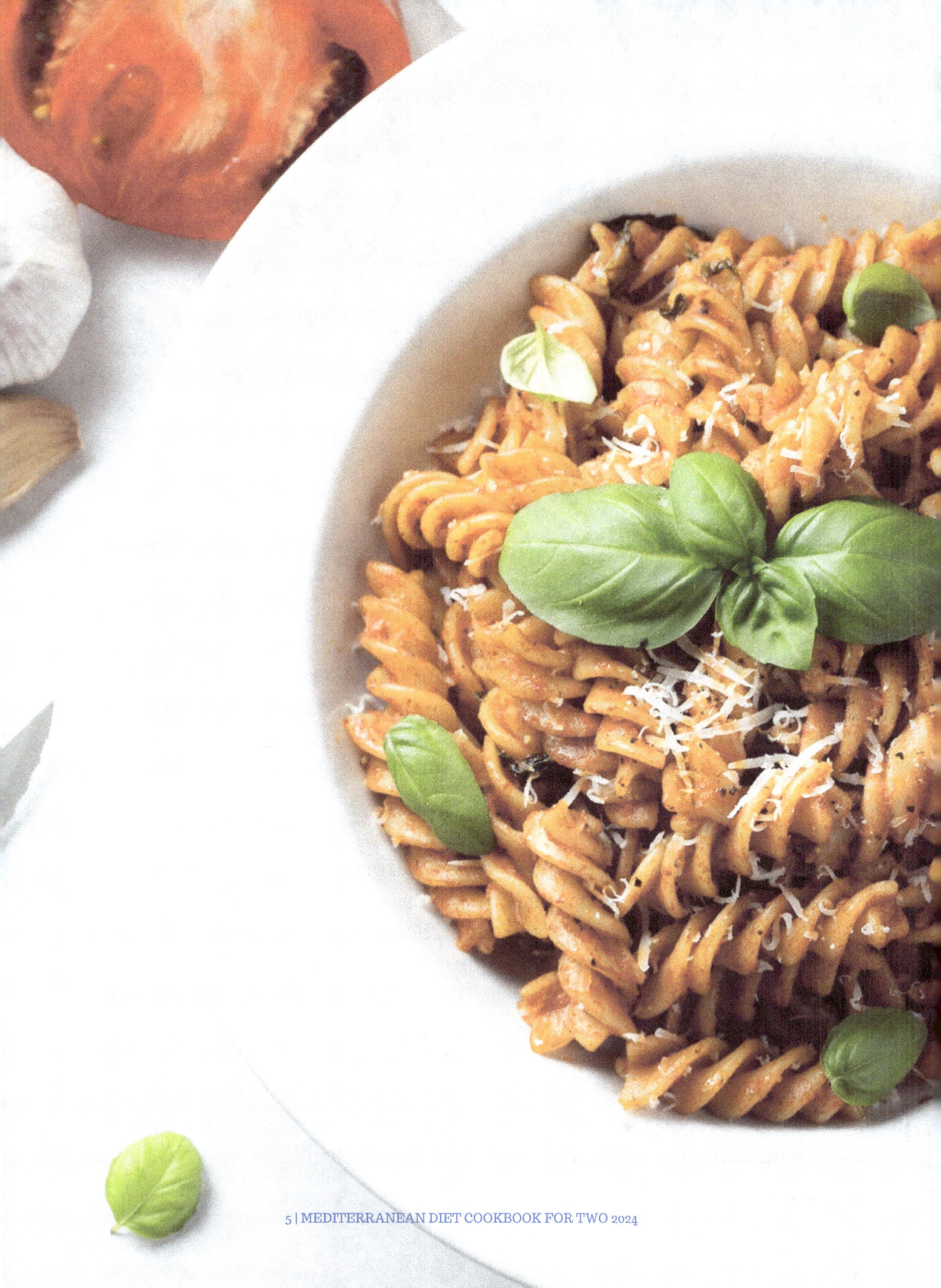

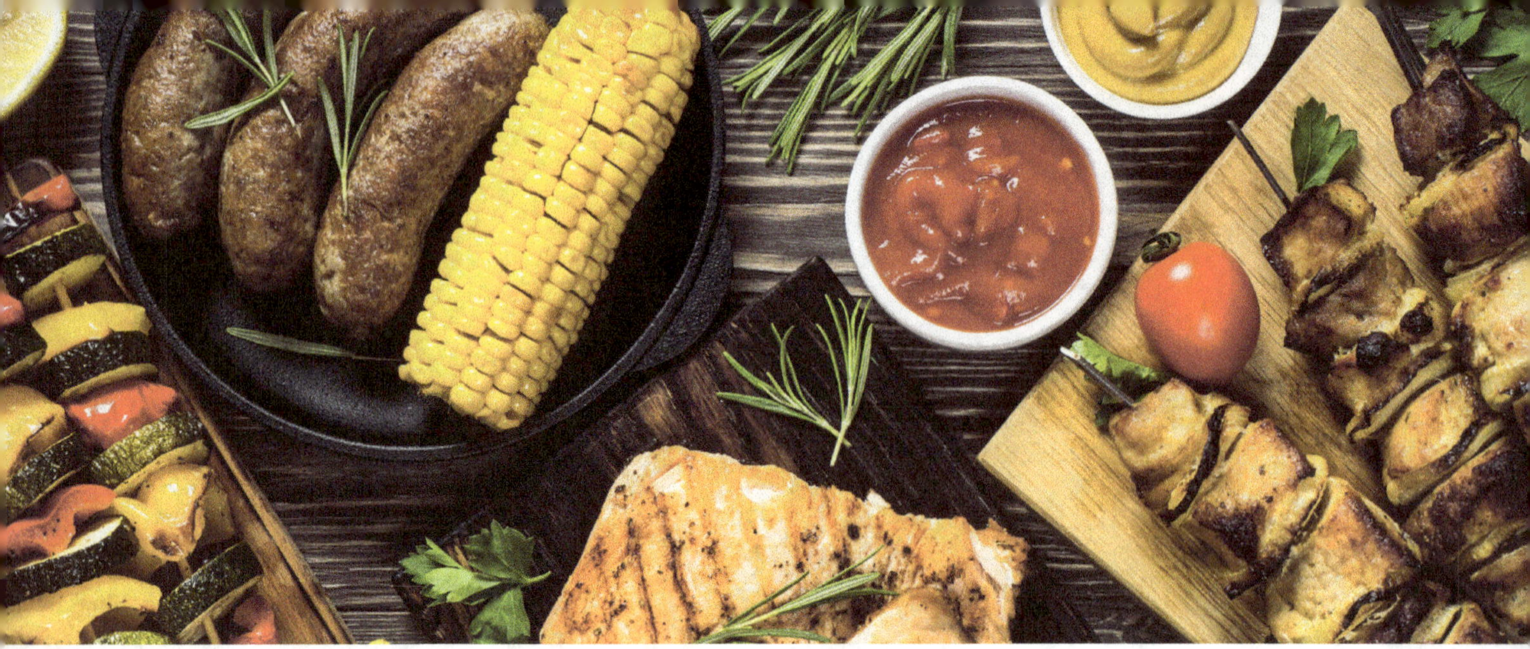

INTRODUCTION

The Mediterranean diet, which is based on the eating habits of southern European nations like Greece, Crete, and Italy, is not only among the tastiest but also among the healthiest. Regardless of food intake, people in these nations often have slim bodies, excellent health, and long, fulfilling lives. Of course, there are a lot of elements that contribute to it (including nature and DNA), but generally speaking, your overall health, appearance, and emotional state are mostly determined by the food you eat.

Whole grains, fresh fruits and vegetables, nuts, olive oil, and fish are the key components of the Mediterranean diet. A minimal amount of meat is consumed. However, it's not just about what you eat—it's also about how you eat it. These days, people don't have as much time to sit down and enjoy their meals, much less spend it with their family and enjoying lunch or supper for an extended period of time.

This diet yields the finest effects when combined with appropriate physical activity: a toned and healthy physique, a positive outlook, and most importantly, a sense of wonderful skin.

The mediterranean diet is an expression of self-love, a way of life. It will not only help you shed the excess weight but also improve your overall health and internal organs.

This diet is one that you may stick to for as long as you choose, unlike any other diet. Making the move to it not too hard, and it will keep you satisfied after every meal. Eating delightful foods—that is, fresh diet is the best approach to lose weight. There won't be protracted bouts of starvation, no need to wean oneself off of delectable meals, and no crankiness brought on by hunger. If your objectives are to get healthy and lose weight without gaining it back, then this diet is worth considering.

Your eating habits will change for the better if you follow the Mediterranean Diet. An important aspect of this diet is to look forward to your next meal and enjoy your meals. I have no doubt that anybody who follows this diet would find the meals enjoyable. The fact that it is full of tasty yet healthful ingredients is what matters.

That is the reason it is adored and well-liked. You'll become more aware of the foods you consume, their freshness, and the components they contain once you start this diet. The most crucial step in becoming a happier, fitter, and healthier person is practicing mindful eating.

Hence, the purpose of this book is to introduce and guide you through the process of beginning a Mediterranean diet. Together, we'll discover why it's so beneficial to your health, if it may help you lose weight, and which foods are best for you.

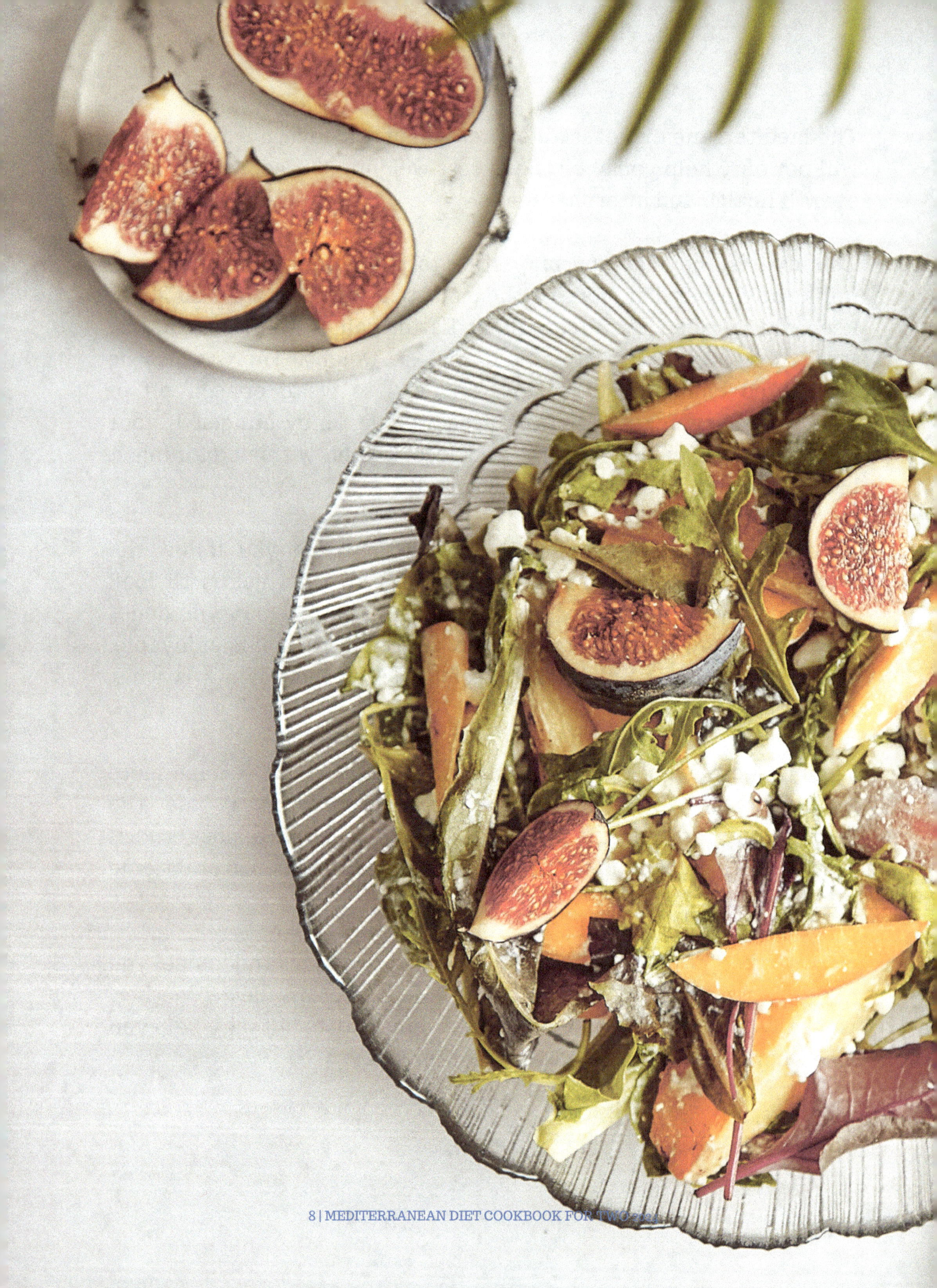

PART I

The Magical Lifestyle Of The Mediterranean

You may be wondering what the key to the health and fitness of Mediterranean people is. The reason for this isn't far-fetched: they consume a lot of whole, fresh food. Their food is usually composed of fruits and vegetables. You would acknowledge that some of the tastiest Mediterranean dishes are really basic, consisting just of veggies and olive oil.

Consuming a diet rich in fruits, vegetables, seafood, nuts, and healthful oils can help your body cleanse itself of all the unnatural elements you were consuming from junk food and fast food. You may easily lose weight if you provide your body the right kinds of nutrients, including proteins, healthy fats, vitamins, minerals, and a fair quantity of carbs.

Furthermore, you would lower your chances of developing diabetes, high cholesterol, heart problems, and cancer. Whole grains, fish, almonds, olive oil, and other healthy fats, along with occasional modest servings of red meat, are the mainstays of the Mediterranean diet. So, how does it function?

The most important aspect of this diet is that it advocates slowing down when you eat, cooking your own food, and spending time with your family. By doing this, you may focus on the tastes and cooking techniques of your dish. You can do this with any diet, of course, but this one excludes all processed foods. Nothing has extra ingredients or additional sweeteners to preserve the food's freshness.

Fresh and full fruits and vegetables (collected from the tree and ground and brought to your table) are included in your meals. Lean meats like fish, olive oil, nutritious grains, lentils, and almost no processed or sugary foods would also be consumed. By giving your body such high-quality foods, you may help it acquire what it needs without storing fat that will go to waste.

Your body stores fat and utilizes carbohydrates for energy when you eat unhealthy meals high in fat and carbs. This is why your arms, legs, and stomach are surrounded by layers of fat.

With a clean and healthy diet, your body gets to use the healthy ingredients, and to burn the fats (since there are no high amounts of carbs in your diet, your body seeks the second best energy source, which is the fat). If you decide to start exercising, your diet will show even better results. The most important thing, I believe you would love, is that this diet is not encouraging you to starve or skip meals.

Every meal is important, and every meal must contain healthy ingredients. You would start your day with a light breakfast. Sure, a light meal will not keep you full for a long time, so instead of going for a snack, you should get a piece of fruit such as berries, a banana, a pear, or whatever fruit you like. Your lunch is the next meal that includes plenty of vegetables combined with healthy fats such as olive oil, cheese, and nuts, and you would finish your day with a dish that contains fish and vegetables, and a glass of red wine.

Following this diet will not stop you from eating foods that have carbohydrates. In this diet, carbs are welcomed. After all, those delicious pasta dishes combined with cooked sauce are people's favorite. Carbohydrates are not your enemy if they are consumed in the right amount and combined with healthy fats (seafood, fish, olive oil), and vegetables.

They are only bad for your weight if it is the only thing you are eating and in large amounts without providing your body with healthy fats, proteins, vitamins, and minerals. As I mentioned, a large amount of carbs helps the body focus on burning the carbs only so it can crate glucose which is the brain's main energy source. The good thing about this diet is that it is so abundant, that you can pick any recipe you want.

Thankfully, this book has loads of nutritious and healthy recipes for you to explore.

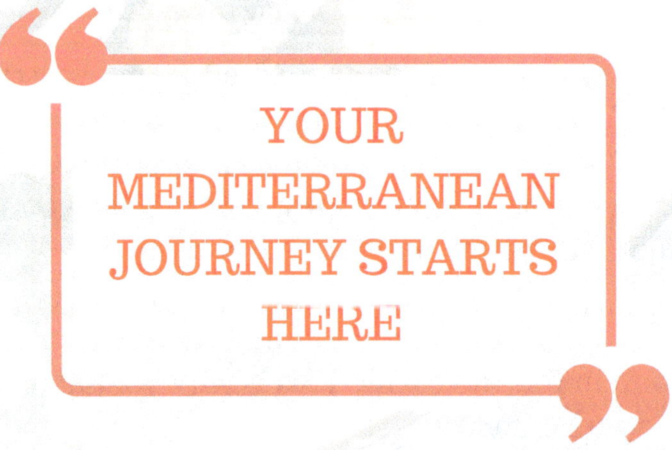

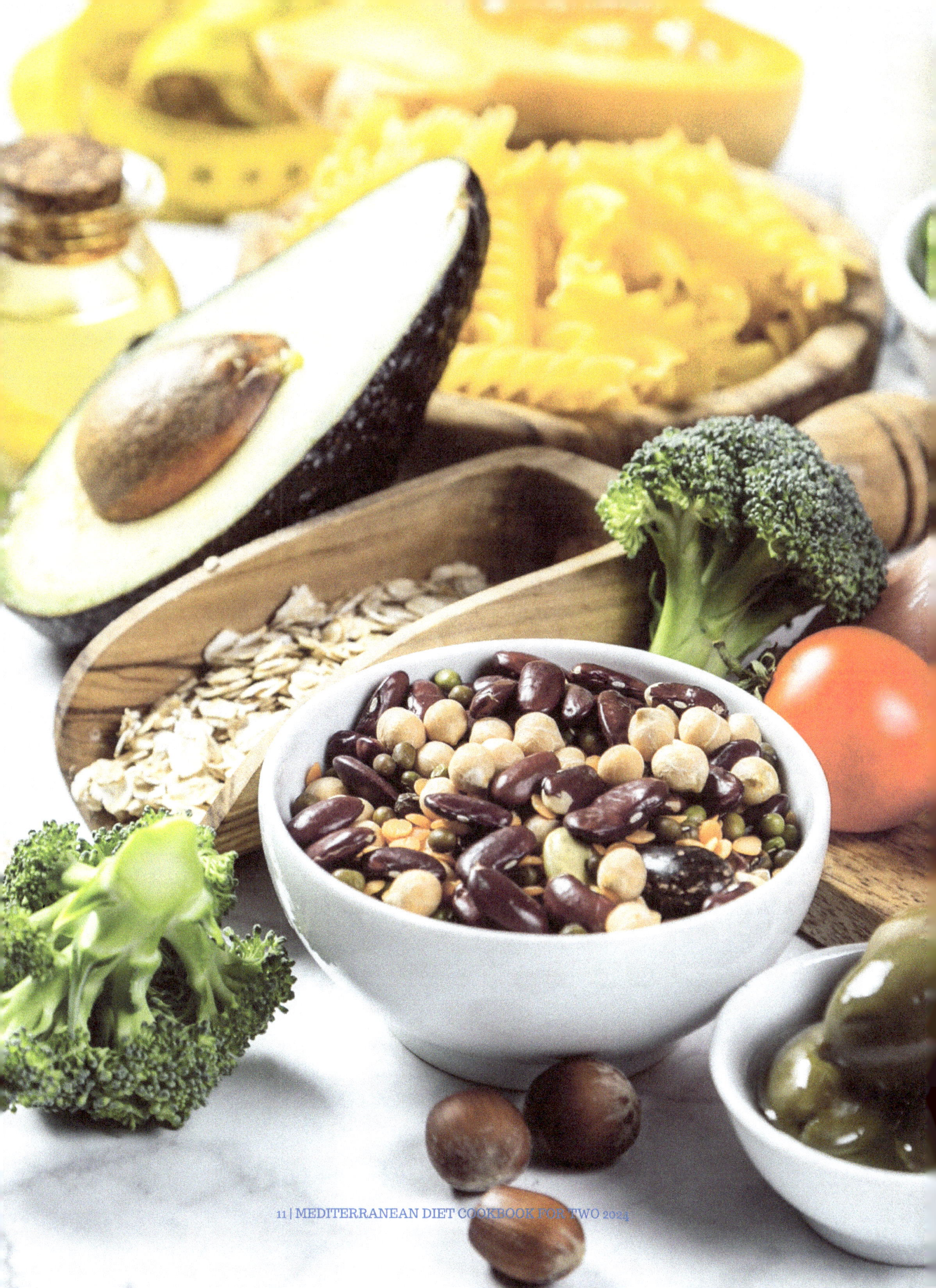

Foods To Eat And Avoid

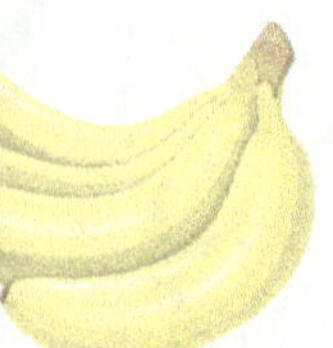

In a Mediterranean-style diet, the following foods are given priority:

- Numerous fresh fruit and vegetable varieties
- Complete grains
- Legumes
- Nuts, seeds, olive oil, and fatty fish are examples of healthy fats.
- A moderate quantity of seafood
- Minimal consumption of dairy and red meat
- Red wine in moderation goes well with meals, but individuals may keep hydrated by drinking water and sugar-free drinks like sparkling water and fresh juice.
- Snacks: When adhering to a Mediterranean diet plan, make an effort to choose snacks that are crafted with wholesome components.

Here are several choices:

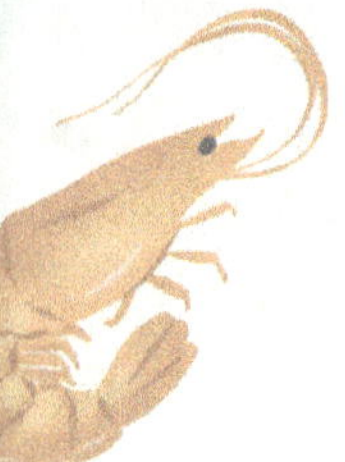

- Fresh fruit and a small amount of nuts together
- Greek yogurt without sugar topped with sunflower seeds and fresh berries
- Fresh veggies and hummus
- Nut and unsweetened dried fruit combined to create a trail mix
- Roasted chickpeas with herb
- Berries with cottage cheese
- A hard-boiled egg, fresh fruit, and a little amount of cheese

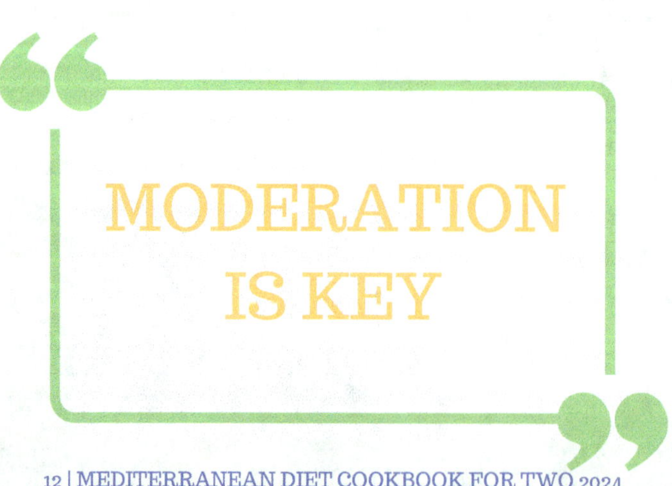

Foods To Restrict Or Steer Away From

Any healthy eating plan, including the Mediterranean diet, should aim to limit your intake of the following foods:

-
- Refined grains, including white flour used in pizza dough, white bread, and white pasta
- Trans fats, found in processed foods like margarine,
- Foods like candy, drinks, and pastries that have added sugar
- Hot dogs, deli meats, and more processed foods
- Highly processed meals, such as fast food

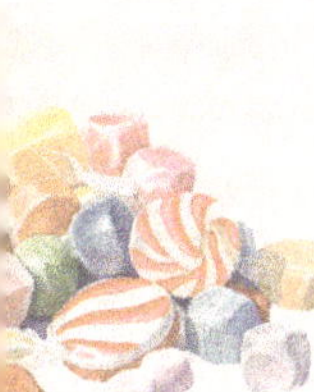

Juicy Health Benefits

The fact that the Mediterranean diet is supported by science is its greatest advantage. Plenty of fruits, vegetables, nuts, seafood, and olive oil are all part of a classic Mediterranean diet, along with suggested physical activity. You may maintain your physical and emotional well-being by following this diet.

1: Lowers the chance of cardiac disorders

A number of studies have shown that a Mediterranean diet may help lower the risk of heart disease, including heart attacks and strokes. You may improve your heart health by eating more fruits, vegetables, olive oil, wine, and whole grains while avoiding red meat, processed foods, and refined sugar. This is known as the Mediterranean diet. In addition to lowering the chance of elevated blood pressure, this diet helps to maintain healthy cholesterol levels.

2: Tonic for the brain

Our body's hungry organ is the brain. Your brain needs a robust blood flow in order to get all of the nutrients and oxygen it needs. Thus, for optimal supply, make sure every vitamin in your diet is good for the brain. This may be satisfied by eating a Mediterranean diet, which also gives your body and brain the nutrition they need. The health of your brain is enhanced by all those good fats, vitamins, and minerals. Additionally, the treatment of anxiety and depression depends heavily on this Mediterranean diet.

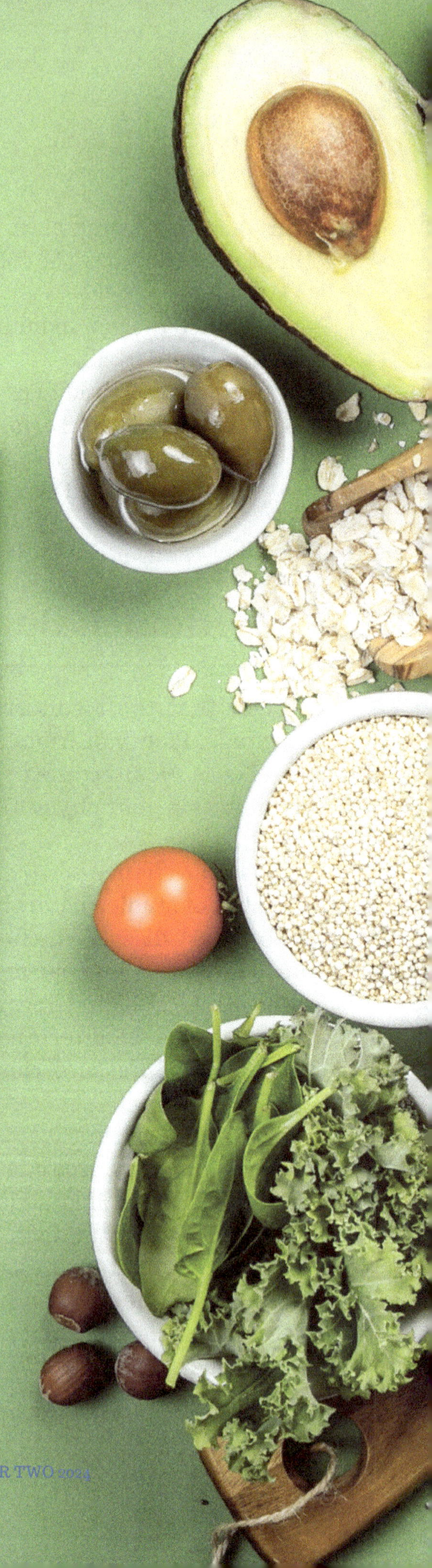
Mediterranean
Diet
meats
sweets
eggs, cheese
poultry
fish, seafood
olive oil
fruits
vegetables
whole
grains
Daily Physical Activity

3. Lowers the chance of Alzheimer's illness

The Mediterranean diet has been shown in several trials to be very effective in lowering the risk of Alzheimer's disease and memory loss. Additionally, this diet helps to lower blood sugar, and cholesterol, and enhance the general health of blood vessels.

4: Encourages responsible weight control

Fiber-rich Mediterranean diets aid in maintaining a healthy weight. Higher-fiber meals make you feel more satisfied and aid in a healthy metabolism and weight reduction. For greater effects, swap out meals high in carbohydrates with foods high in fiber, such as nuts and veggies.

5. Prevents Diabetes

Many fibers included in a Mediterranean diet slow down digestion, stabilize blood sugar levels, and aid in maintaining a healthy weight. According to research, a Mediterranean diet may also enhance the body's capacity to use insulin.

6. Lowers the chance of developing cancer

A Mediterranean diet lowers the chance of developing some types of cancer. Research indicates that consuming a Mediterranean diet may strengthen your immune system, making you more resistant to diseases like breast and colon cancer. It can also reduce your risk of dying from cancer.

7. Alleviates Rheumatoid Arthritic Pain

An autoimmune condition that causes joint discomfort and swelling is called rheumatoid arthritis (RA). Omega-3 fatty acids, which have anti-inflammatory properties and may help reduce RA symptoms, are abundant in the Mediterranean diet.

KEY TAKEAWAY

Based on the customs of Mediterranean nations, the Mediterranean diet is a healthful eating regimen. This diet urges us to reduce processed meals and sweets and to consume healthful foods rich in vitamins, fiber, minerals, and fatty acids. Numerous health advantages stem from this heart-healthy Mediterranean diet, including the prevention of serious illnesses like cancer.

Making sustainable, long-term food decisions is a need of the Mediterranean diet. It is a diet high in whole grains, veggies, and healthy fats. However, a nutritionist should be consulted by anybody who feels that the diet is not fulfilling. To aid in boosting fullness, they might suggest more or different meals.

meal plan
1 Day
2 Day
3 Day

PART II
Mediterranean 14-day meal plan

All recipes have been covered in detail in the book

Day 1:
Breakfast: Mediterranean Avocado Toast with Poached Eggs
Lunch: Mediterranean Quinoa Salad with Lemon-Herb Vinaigrette
Dinner: Mediterranean Grilled Chicken with Lemon-Herb Quinoa
Snack: Cranberry-Almond Energy Balls

Day 2:
Breakfast: Greek Yogurt Parfait with Honey and Nuts
Lunch: Mediterranean Chickpea and Spinach Stew
Dinner: Mediterranean Baked Salmon with Roasted Vegetables
Snack: Cottage Cheese with Raspberry Honey

Day 3:
Breakfast: Mediterranean Veggie Omelette
Lunch: Greek Chicken Souvlaki Wrap
Dinner: Skillet Lemon-Chicken, Potatoes with Kale
Snack: Cauliflower Hummus

Day 4:
Breakfast: Mediterranean Shakshuka
Lunch: Mediterranean Lentil and Vegetable Stuffed Peppers
Dinner: Mediterranean Lentil Soup with Spinach
Snack: Pretzels with Dark Chocolate & Peanut Butter

Day 5:
Breakfast: Mediterranean Breakfast Wrap
Lunch: Mediterranean Shrimp and Orzo Salad
Dinner: Mediterranean Shrimp Pasta with Tomato-Basil Sauce
Snack: Pineapple Nice Cream

Day 6:
Breakfast: Mediterranean Chia Seed Pudding
Lunch: Mediterranean Hummus and Veggie Wrap
Dinner: Mediterranean Chickpea Salad with Lemon-Tahini Dressing
Snack: No-Sugar-Added Mini Apple Pies

Day 7:
Breakfast: Mediterranean Quinoa Breakfast Bowl
Lunch: Mediterranean Grilled Vegetable and Quinoa Bowl
Dinner: Mediterranean Stuffed Bell Peppers with Ground Turkey
Snack: Cranberry-Almond Energy Balls

Day 8:
Breakfast: Mediterranean Egg and Spinach Breakfast Sandwich
Lunch: Mediterranean Stuffed Portobello Mushrooms
Dinner: Mediterranean Veggie Pita Wrap with Tzatziki

Snack: Cottage Cheese with Raspberry Honey

Day 9:
Breakfast: Mediterranean Breakfast Couscous Bowl
Lunch: Mediterranean Turkey and Vegetable Skewers
Dinner: Mediterranean Eggplant and Chickpea Bake
Snack: Pretzels with Dark Chocolate & Peanut Butter

Day 10:
Breakfast: Mediterranean Smashed Chickpea Toast
Lunch: Mediterranean Farro Salad with Roasted Vegetables
Dinner: Mediterranean Baked Salmon with Roasted Vegetables
Snack: Pineapple Nice Cream

Day 11:
Breakfast: Greek Yogurt Parfait with Honey and Nuts
Lunch: Mediterranean Lentil and Vegetable Stuffed Peppers
Dinner: Skillet-Lemon Chicken & Potatoes with Kale
Snack: No-Sugar-Added Mini Apple Pies

Day 12:
Breakfast: Mediterranean Veggie Omelette
Lunch: Mediterranean Shrimp and Orzo Salad
Dinner: Mediterranean Chickpea Salad with Lemon-Tahini Dressing
Snack: Cranberry-Almond Energy Balls

Day 13:
Breakfast: Mediterranean Chia Seed Pudding
Lunch: Mediterranean Grilled Vegetable and Quinoa Bowl
Dinner: Mediterranean Stuffed Bell Peppers with Ground Turkey
Snack: Cottage Cheese with Raspberry Honey

Day 14:
Breakfast: Mediterranean Quinoa Breakfast Bowl
Lunch: Mediterranean Turkey and Vegetable Skewers
Dinner: Mediterranean Veggie Pita Wrap with Tzatziki
Snack: Pineapple Nice Cream

Feel free to adjust the order of the meals based on your preferences. Additionally, make sure to stay mindful of portion sizes, drink plenty of water, and listen to your body's hunger and fullness cues. This 14-day Mediterranean diet meal plan is designed to provide a variety of nutrients while offering delicious and satisfying meals. Enjoy your culinary journey!

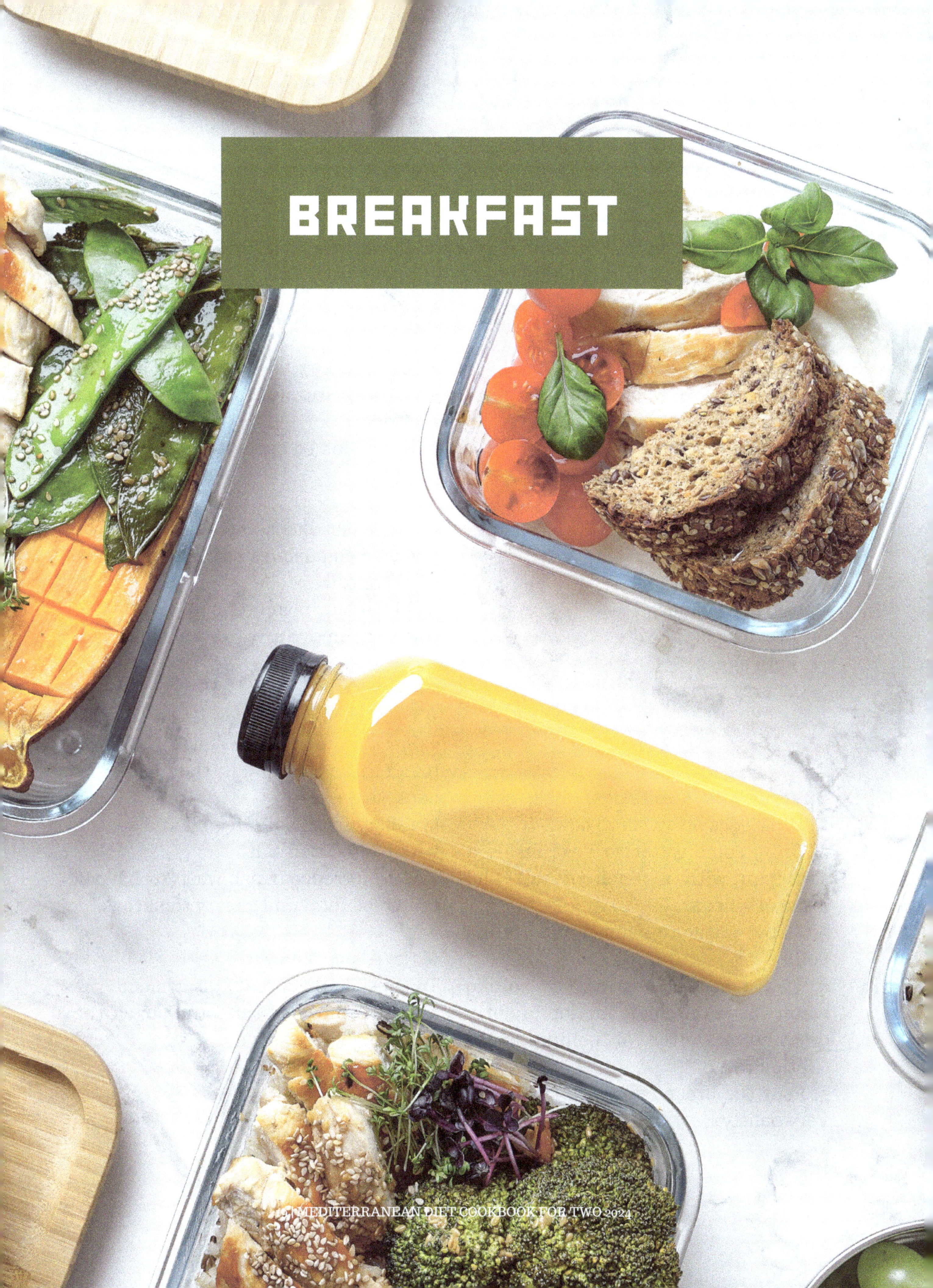
BREAKFAST

Mediterranean Avocado Toast with Poached Eggs

A delicious take on the traditional avocado toast, this Mediterranean variation amps up the protein content with poached eggs.

 Cooking/Prep Time: 15 mins 🍽 Servings: 2

Ingredients

- Two pieces of wholegrain bread
- One ripe avocado
- Four big eggs
- One tablespoon of olive oil
- Spice with salt and pepper

Optional Toppings::

- Fresh basil
- Feta cheese
- Cherry tomatoes

Directions To Poach Egg

1. Break eggs into a small bowl.
2. Bring some water to heat inside a saucepan with a pinch of salt and some of vinegar.
3. Allow water to simmer not rolling boil.
4. Use a spoon to swirl the boiling water in a circular motion, gently creating a vortex of boiling water (Optional).
5. Pour the broken egg into the water very gently.
6. Let the egg white solidify and the yolk stay runny for three to four minutes.
7. Use a slotted spoon to take eggs out of water.

8. Take out excess moisture from the poached egg using a soft kitchen towel or paper towel.
9. Place the poached egg on a paper towel to remove any excess liquid.

Directions

1. Toast the bread slices.
2. Spread the avocado equally over the bread after mashing it, then place the eggs.
3. Add a drizzle of olive oil and season with pepper and salt.
4. If preferred, garnish with fresh basil, crumbled feta, and cherry tomatoes.

Make Ahead Tips

To speed up breakfast, mash the avocado ahead of time and poach the eggs just before serving.

Nutritional Value (Per Serving)

Calories: 320 | Carbs: 22g | Protein: 14g | Fats: 20g | Fiber: 7g

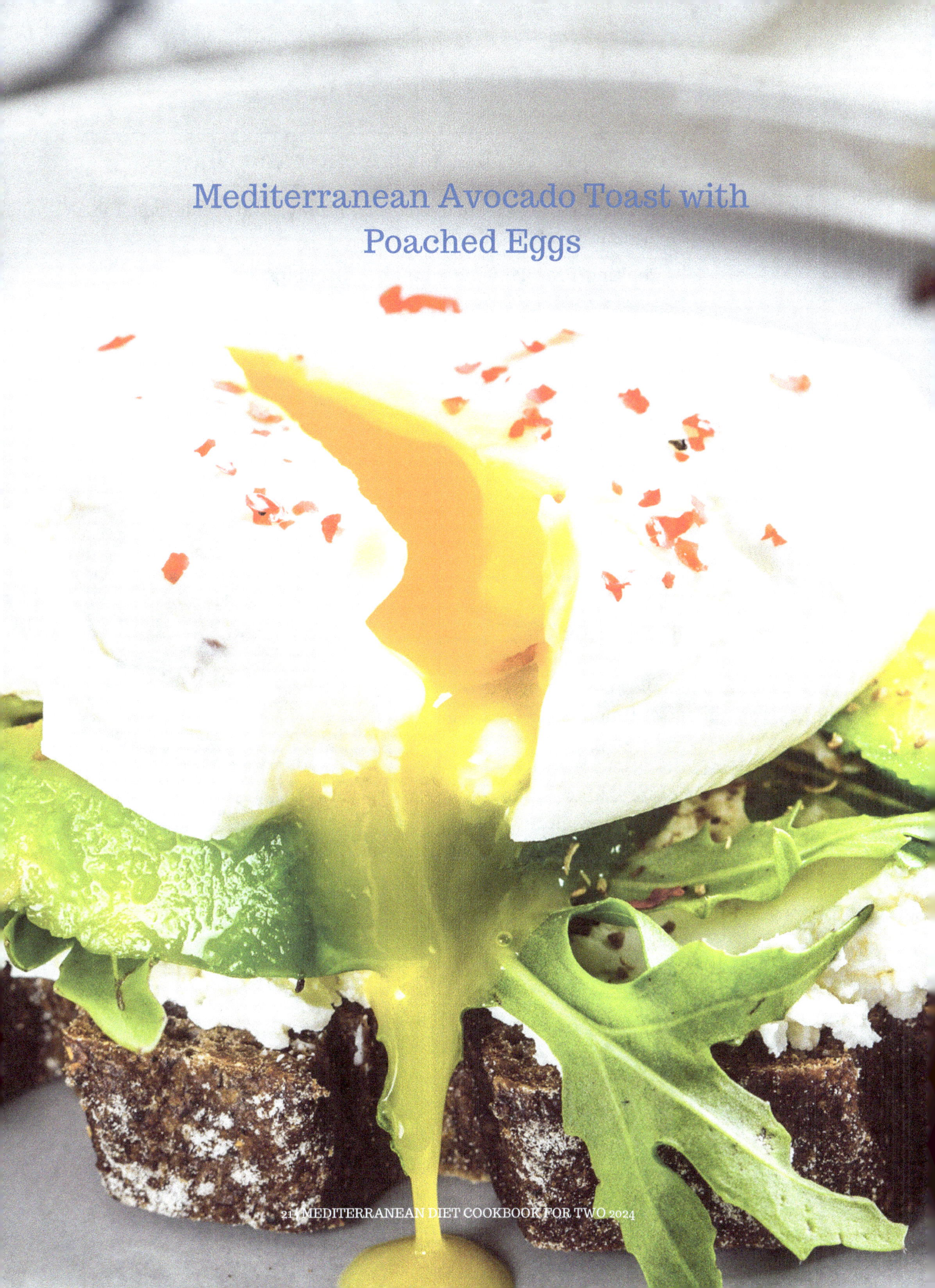
Mediterranean Avocado Toast with
Poached Eggs

Greek Yogurt Parfait with Honey and Nuts

A rich Greek yogurt parfait topped with almonds, honey, and fresh fruit for a wholesome and revitalizing start to the day.

Cooking/Prep Time: 10 mins   Servings: 2

Ingredients

- Two cups of Greek yogurt
- Four tsp honey
- 1/2 cup of mixed nuts, such as pistachios, walnuts, or almonds
- One cup of mixed berries, either blueberries, raspberries, or strawberries

DIRECTIONS:

1. Arrange Greek yogurt, fruit, honey, and almonds in two glasses.
2. Layers should be repeated until the glasses are full.
3. Sprinkle the uppermost layer with honey and add more almonds.

MAKE AHEAD/COOKING HINTS:

To make a speedy breakfast, prepare the parfait the night before and refrigerate.

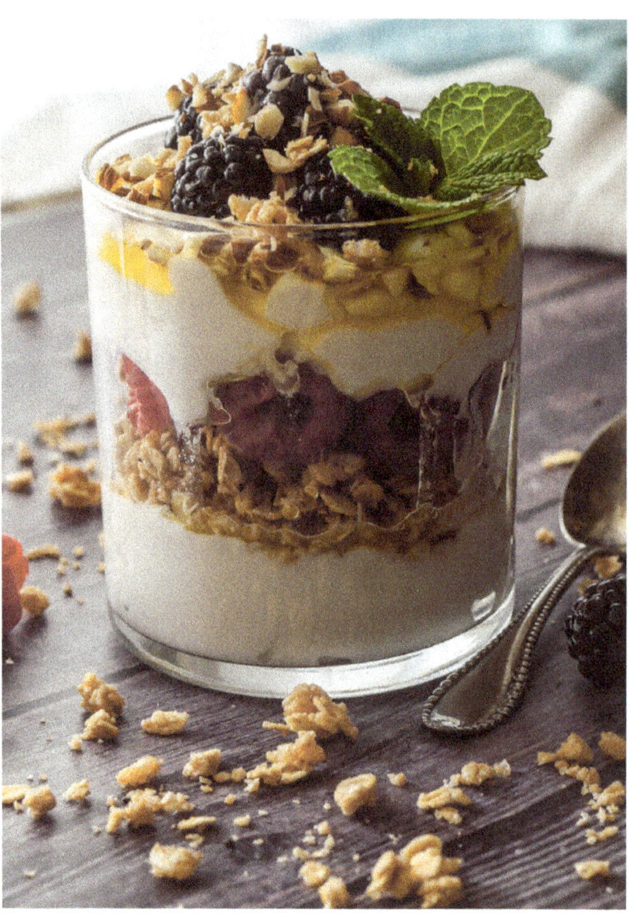

Nutritional Value (Per Serving)

Calories: 380 | Carbs: 30g | Protein: 18g | Fats: 22g | Fiber: 6g

Mediterranean Veggie Omelette

This omelette, loaded with feta cheese and Mediterranean veggies, is a flavorful and filling morning dish.

 Cooking/Prep Time: 20 mins 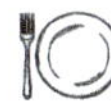 Servings: 2

Ingredients

- Four big eggs
- One tablespoon of olive oil
- Half a red bell pepper, chopped
- Half a red onion, cut finely;
- One small zucchini, sliced; one diced tomato
- 1/4 cup of feta cheese, crumbled
- Fresh herbs, such as oregano or parsley
- Salt and pepper.

Directions

1. In a bowl, whip eggs and add pepper and salt as needed.
2. In a skillet with heated olive oil, sauté the peppers, onions, and zucchini until they are soft.
3. Over the vegetables, pour the whisked eggs and let to set slightly.
4. Top one side of the omelette with fresh herbs, feta, and tomatoes.
5. After folding the second half over the contents, cook the eggs until they are set through.

NUTRITIONAL VALUE (PER SERVING):

Calories: 280 Carbs: 9g Protein: 18g Fats: 20g Fiber: 3g

Make Ahead Tips

To expedite the morning preparation, prepare the chopped vegetables the night before.

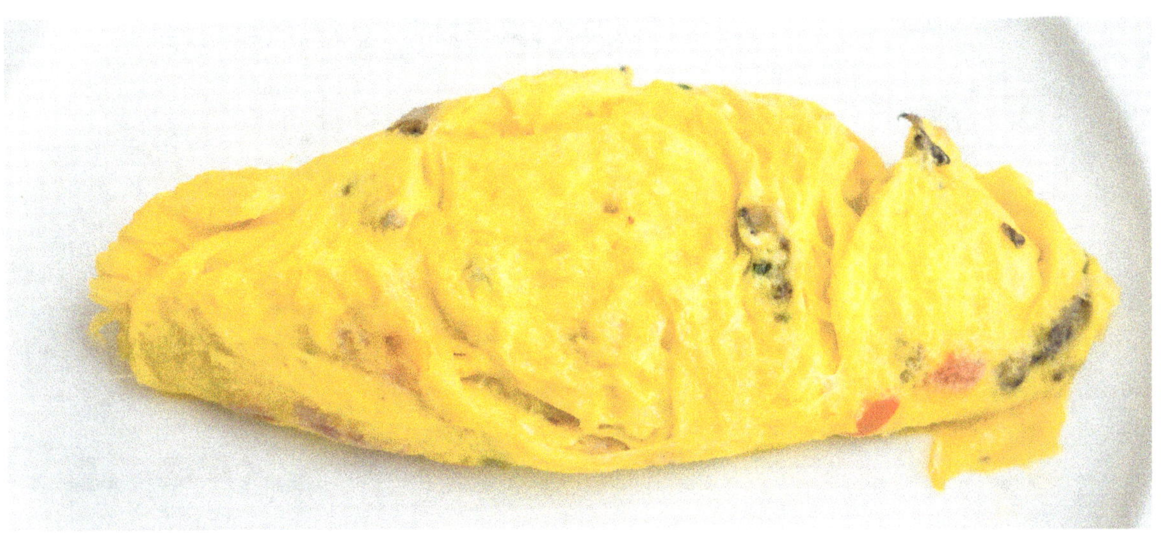

Mediterranean Shakshuka

A rich and savory breakfast dish with poached eggs in a sauce made with tomatoes and bell peppers and seasoned with paprika and cumin.

Cooking/Prep Time: 25 mins | Servings: 2

Ingredients

- Four big eggs
- One tablespoon of olive oil
- One onion, chopped finely
- Two chopped bell peppers, red and yellow
- 2 minced garlic cloves
- One can, or fourteen ounces of chopped tomatoes
- One teaspoon of cumin
- One tsp of paprika
- Season with salt and pepper and Add fresh parsley as a garnish.

Directions

1. In a skillet with heated olive oil, fry till soften onions, garlic, and bell peppers.
2. Add the paprika, cumin, chopped tomatoes, salt, and pepper. Simmer for ten to fifteen minutes.
3. In the sauce, make wells and break eggs into them.
4. Cover and poach eggs in the simmering sauce until the whites are set but the yolks are still runny.
5. Before serving, garnish with fresh parsley.

NUTRITIONAL VALUE (PER SERVING):

Calories: 320 | Carbs: 18g | Protein: 16g | Fats: 22g | Fiber: 4g

COOKING AND PREPARATION TIP:

To expedite the morning preparation, prepare the chopped vegetables the night before.

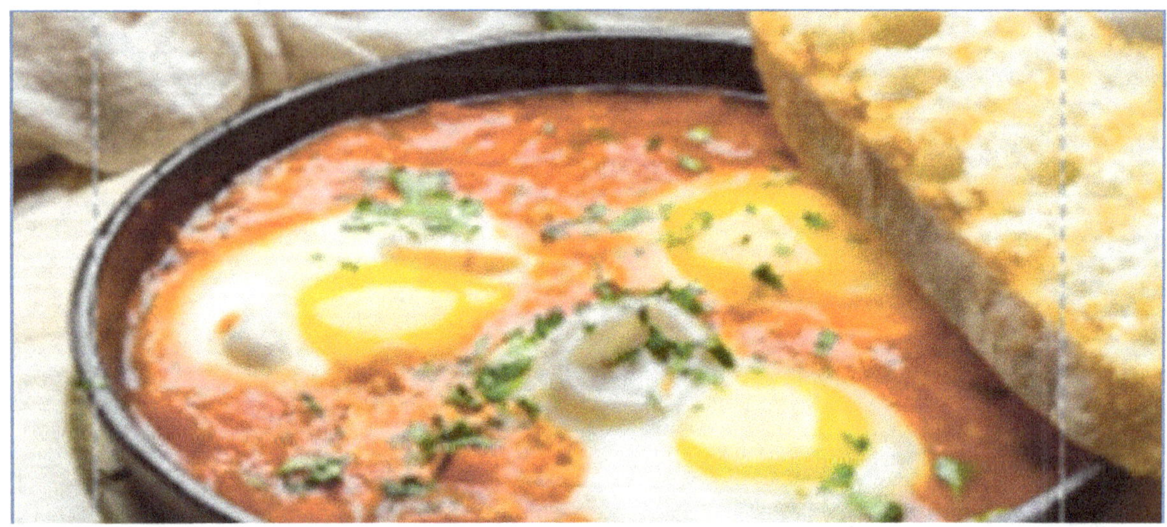

Mediterranean Breakfast Wrap

A lightweight, wholesome breakfast sandwich stuffed with sun-dried tomatoes, feta, spinach, and scrambled eggs.

 Cooking/Prep Time: 15 mins 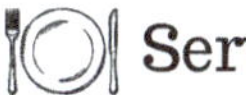 Servings: 2

Ingredients

- Four big scrambled eggs
- Two wraps made with healthy grains
- One cup of raw spinach
- 1/2 cup of feta cheese, crumbled
- 1/4 cup chopped sun-dried tomatoes
- Add seasoning to taste.

Directions

1. Cook the eggs in a pan, scrambling them, and season with salt and pepper.
2. Use a microwave or a dry skillet to reheat the wraps.
3. Divide the sun-dried tomatoes, feta, spinach, and scrambled eggs evenly among the wraps.
4. After folding the sides, then roll them up.

NUTRITIONAL VALUE (PER SERVING):

Calories: 340 | Carbs: 26g | Protein: 20g | Fats: 18g | Fiber: 6g

MAKE AHEAD/COOKING TIPS:

Cut the vegetables and make the scrambled eggs ahead of time for fast assembling.

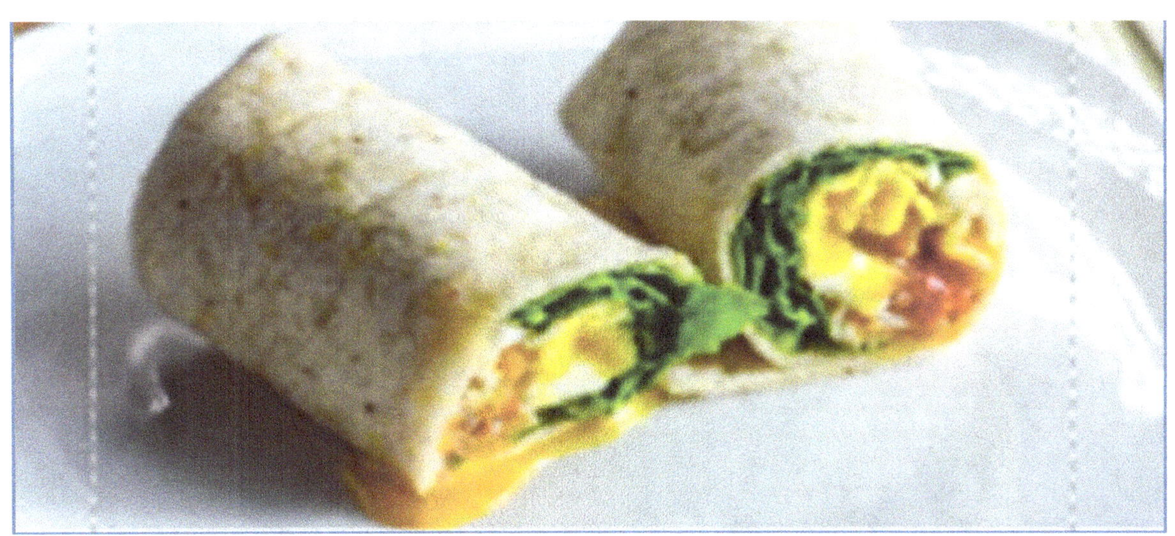

Mediterranean Chia Seed Pudding

A filling and healthy chia seed pudding with Mediterranean tastes, garnished with almonds and fresh fruit.

 Cooking/Prep Time: 4hrs5 mins 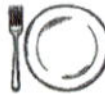 Servings: 2

Ingredients

- A quarter cup of chia seeds
- A cup of almond milk
- A tablespoon of honey
- Half a teaspoon of vanilla extract
- A quarter teaspoon of ground cinnamon
- Fresh fruits (figs, pomegranate seeds) and nuts for topping

NUTRITIONAL VALUE (PER SERVING):

Calories: 250 | Carbs: 28g | Protein: 6g | Fats: 12g | Fiber: 10g

Directions

1. Chia seeds, almond milk, honey, cinnamon, and vanilla essence should all be combined in a bowl.
2. Place the mixture in the refrigerator for four hours or overnight.
3. Mix well and garnish with nuts and fresh fruits just before serving.

MAKE AHEAD/COOKING TIPS:

For an easy morning treat, make the chia seed combination the night before.

Note: The chia pudding is ready in 5 to 10 mins, the 4 hours is for the refrigeration time.

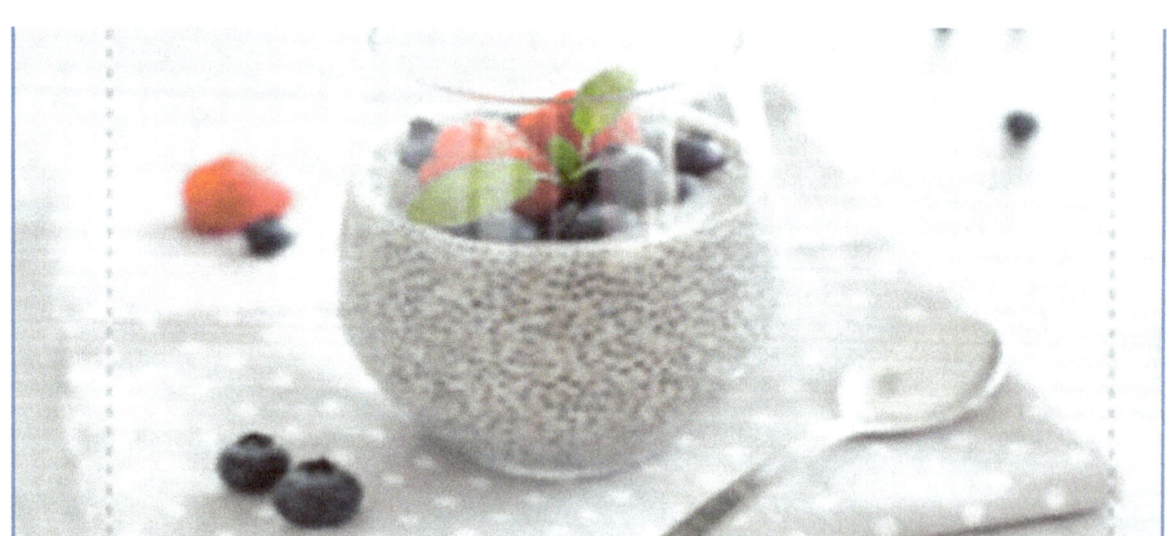

Mediterranean Quinoa Breakfast Bowl

A high-protein breakfast dish with quinoa, fresh fruit, Greek yogurt, and honey drizzled on top.

 Cooking/Prep Time: 15 mins 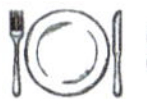 Servings: 2

Ingredients

- Half a cup of cooked quinoa
- One cup of Greek yogurt
- One cup of mixed berries (strawberries and blueberries)
- 1/4 cup of finely chopped nuts (walnuts or almonds)
- Honey

NUTRITIONAL VALUE (PER SERVING):

Calories: 320 | Carbs: 42g | Protein: 15g | Fats: 10g | Fiber: 6g

Directions

1. To cook the quinoa, follow the directions given on the package.
2. Divide the cooked quinoa into two separate bowls.
3. Add chopped nuts, mixed berries, and Greek yogurt on top.
4. Before serving, pour some honey over it.

TIPS:

Prepare the quinoa ahead of time to save time while making breakfast.

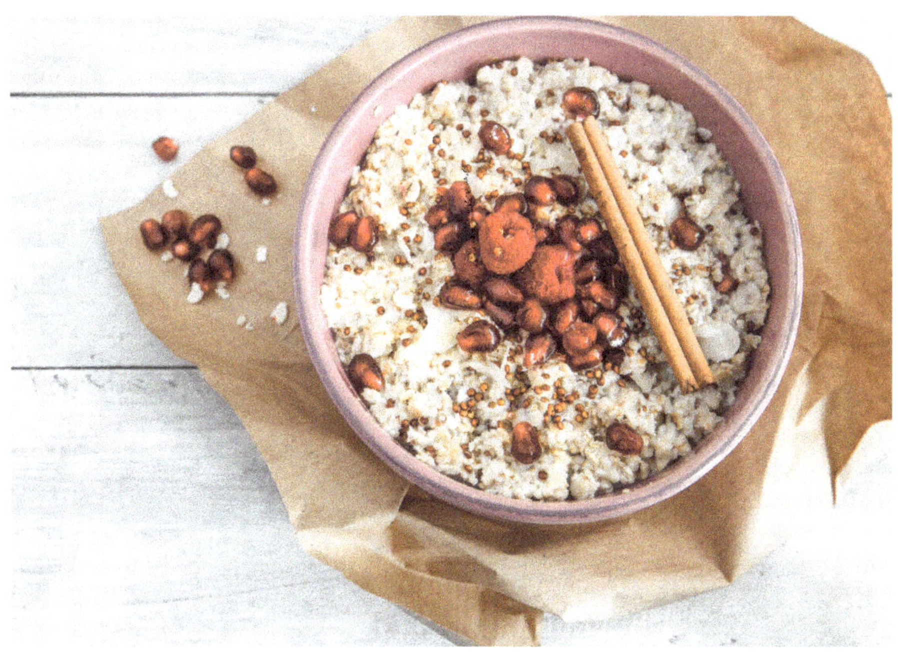

Mediterranean Egg and Spinach Breakfast Sandwich

A healthy breakfast sandwich made with feta cheese, sautéed spinach, and a properly cooked egg served on a whole-grain English muffin.

🕐 Cooking/Prep Time: 15 mins   🍽 Servings: 2

Ingredients

- Two toasted wholegrain English muffins
- Two big eggs
- one cup of raw spinach
- 1/4 cup of feta cheese, crumbled
- Seasoning (Salt and spices)

Directions

1. Season the eggs and cook them to your preference in a skillet.
2. Fresh spinach should be sautéed till it wilst.
3. Gather the sandwiches with the eggs, spinach, and crumbled feta on the toasted English muffins.

NUTRITIONAL VALUE (PER SERVING):

Calories: 280 | Carbs: 30g | Protein: 14g | Fats: 12g | Fiber: 5g

MAKE AHEAD/COOKING TIPS:

Prepare the sautéed spinach in advance for a quicker breakfast assembly.

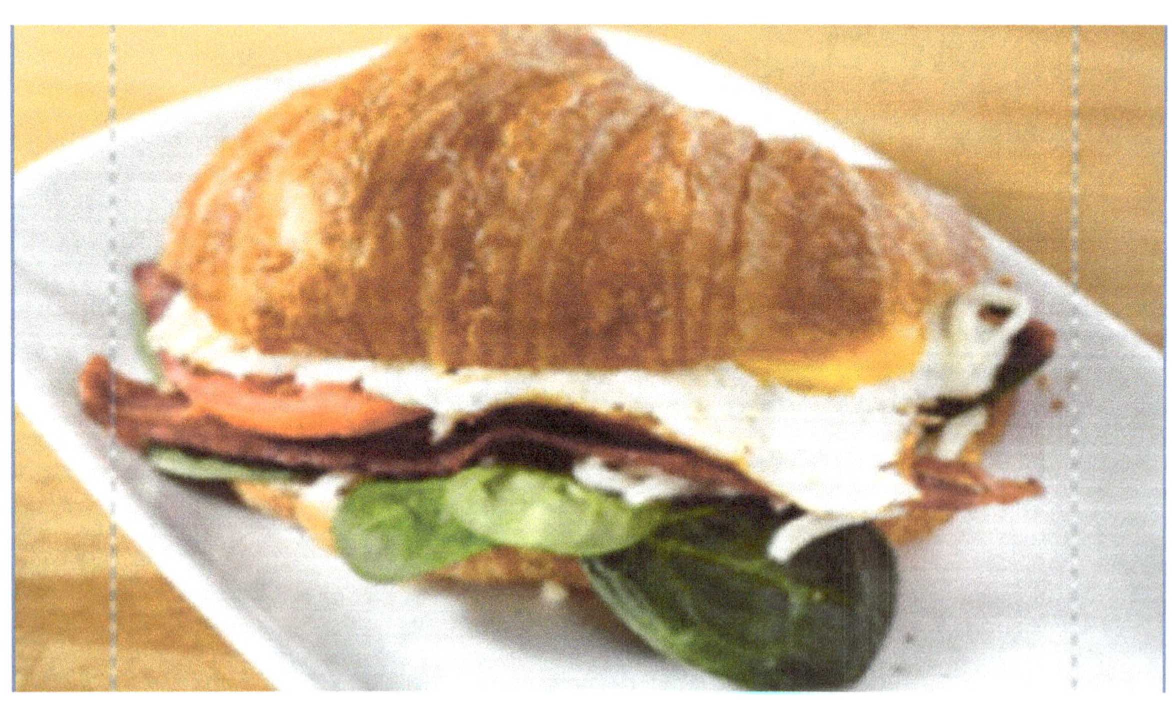

Mediterranean Breakfast Couscous Bowl

A Mediterranean-inspired couscous dish topped with cherry tomatoes, olives, and poached eggs.

 Cooking/Prep Time: 20 mins 🍽 Servings: 2

Ingredients

- A cup of couscous, cooked
- Four large eggs
- One cup of cherry tomatoes, halved
- A quarter cup of Kalamata olives, sliced
- Two tablespoons of fresh parsley, chopped
- 1 tablespoon of olive oil
- Seasonings

Directions

1. Prepare the couscous as directed on the packet.
2. To your preference, poach the eggs.
3. Divide the cooked couscous into two bowls.
4. Add poached eggs, olives, cherry tomatoes, and fresh parsley on top.
5. Add spices and a drizzle of olive oil to taste.

NUTRITIONAL VALUE (PER SERVING):

Calories: 340 | Carbs: 38g | Protein: 17g | Fats: 14g | Fiber: 4g

MAKE AHEAD/COOKING TIPS:

Prepare the couscous and poach the eggs simultaneously for an efficient morning preparation.

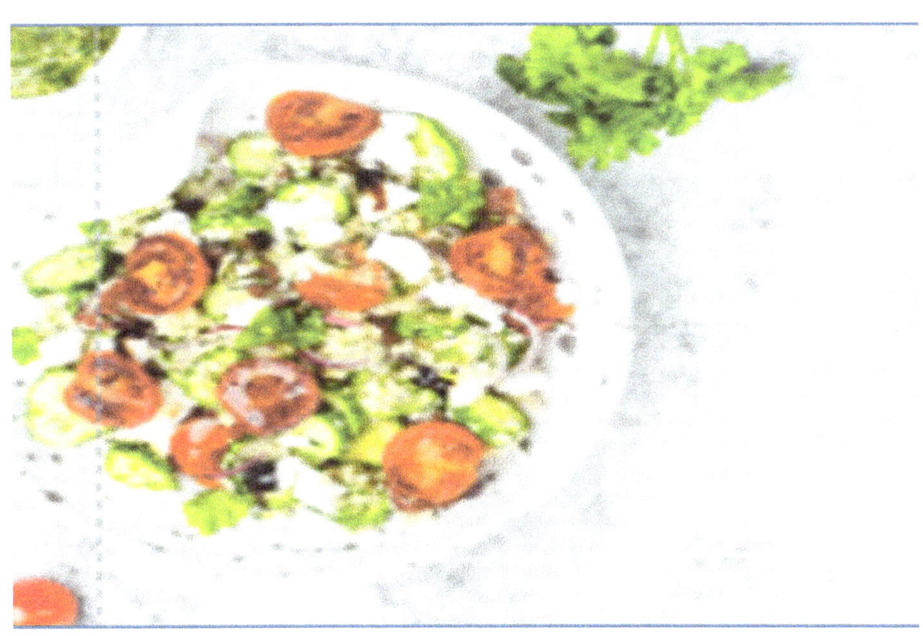

Mediterranean Smashed Chickpea Toast

A delightfully crunchy breakfast with a Mediterranean flair, this protein-packed toast is topped with cherry tomatoes, feta, and crushed chickpeas.

 Cooking/Prep Time: 15 mins   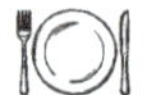 Servings: 2

Ingredients

- Four (4) slices of whole-grain bread and one can (15 oz) of rinsed and drained chickpeas
- One tablespoon of olive oil
- One tablespoon of lemon juice
- 1/4 tsp cumin
- Seasonings
- Cherry tomatoes, sliced
- Feta cheese, crumbled
- Fresh basil leaves for garnish

Directions

1. Smash the chickpeas and combine them with the lemon juice, cumin, olive oil, salt, and pepper in a bowl.
2. Spread pieces of toasted bread with the chickpea mixture.
3. Add fresh basil, crumbled feta, and cherry tomato slices on top.

NUTRITIONAL VALUE (PER SERVING):

Calories: 320 | Carbs: 50g | Protein: 14g | Fats: 10g | Fiber: 12g

MAKE AHEAD/COOKING TIPS:

For a quick breakfast, prepare the crushed chickpea mixture ahead of time.

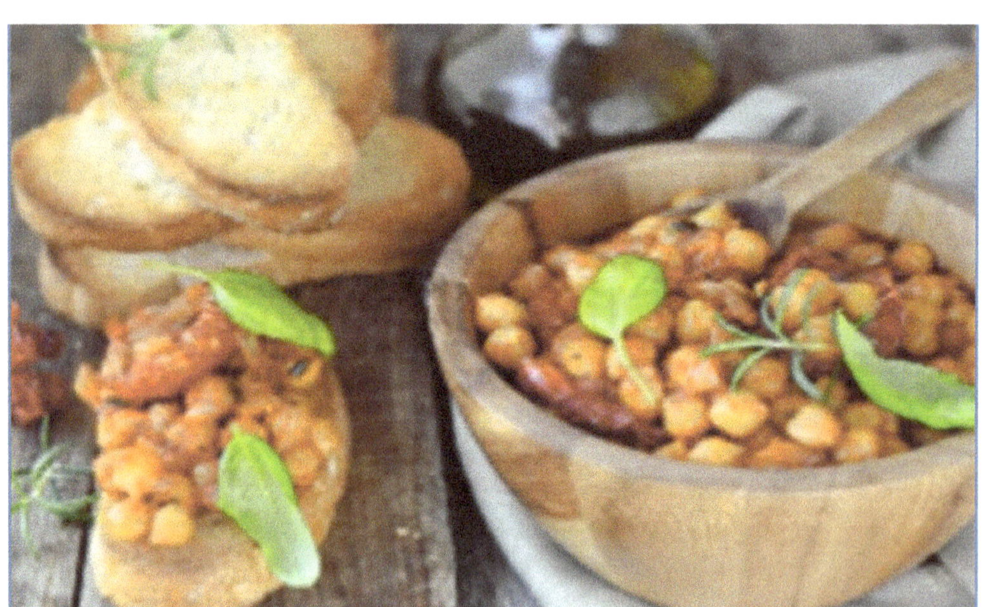

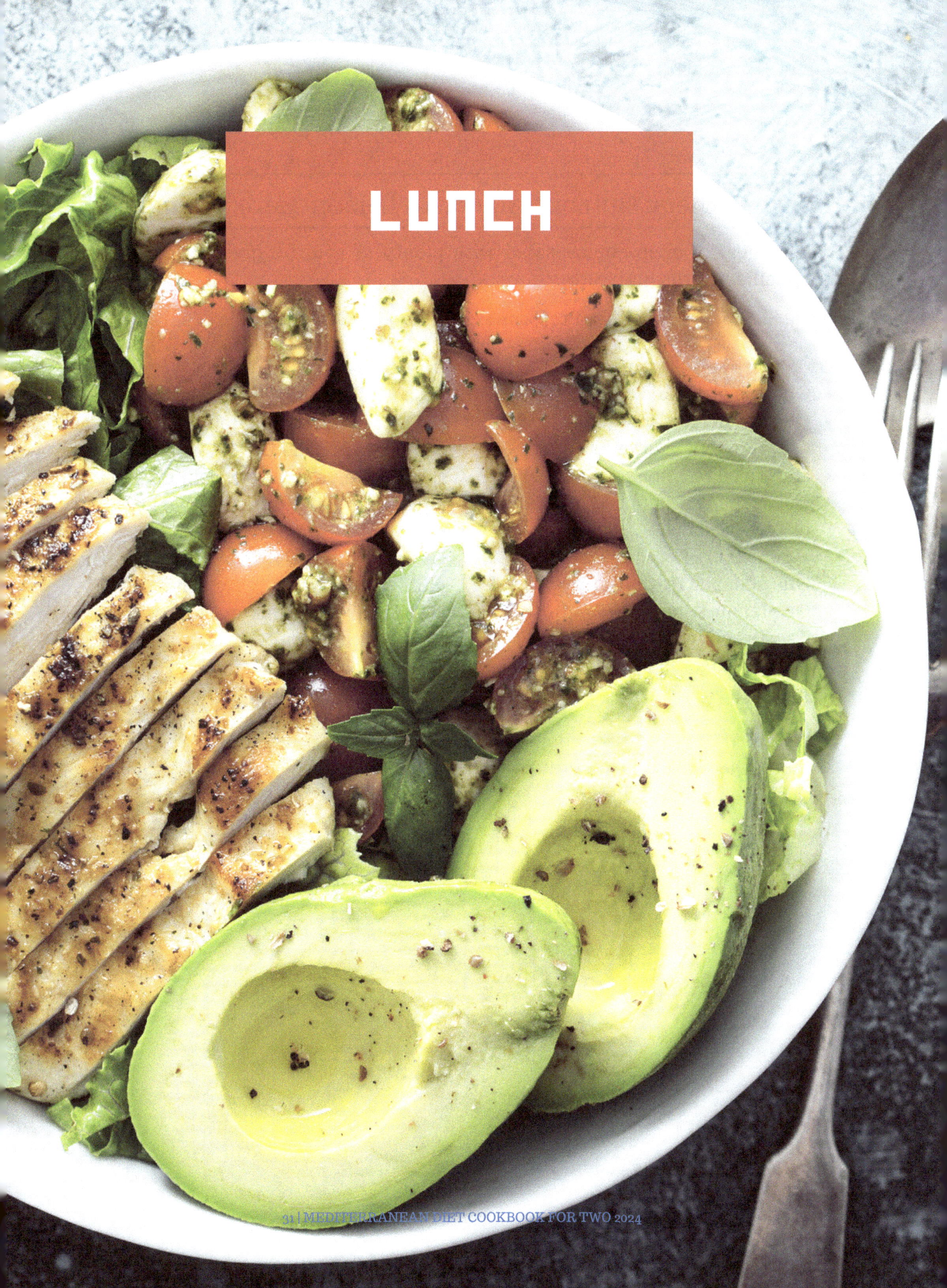

LUNCH

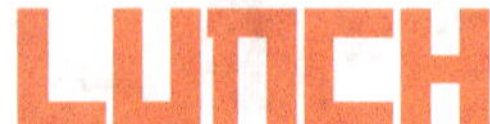

Mediterranean Quinoa Salad with Lemon-Herb Vinaigrette

A light meal of crisp quinoa salad with plenty of colorful greens, feta, and a tangy lemon-herb vinaigrette.

 Cooking/Prep Time: 20 mins 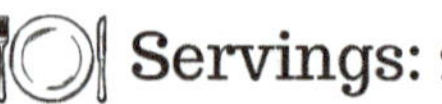 Servings: 2

Ingredients

- One cup of cooked quinoa,
- One cup of cherry tomatoes,
- One cucumber cut in half
- One diced red onion,
- One finely chopped Kalamata olive, one sliced
- 1/4 cup feta cheese
- One chopped fresh parsley
- One lemon's juice
- Two tsp olive oil
- Add seasoning according to preference.

Nutritional Value (Per Serving)

Calories: 380 | Carbs:45g | Protein: 12g | Fats: 18g | Fiber: 7g

Directions

1. Cooked quinoa, cucumber, tomatoes, red onion, olives, and feta should all be combined in a dish.
2. For the vinaigrette, combine lemon juice, olive oil, salt, and pepper in a small container.
3. Over the salad, drizzle with the vinaigrette, mix gently, and sprinkle with the fresh parsley.

Make Ahead Tips

Cook the quinoa ahead for quick meal. Set aside the vinaigrette until ready to serve.

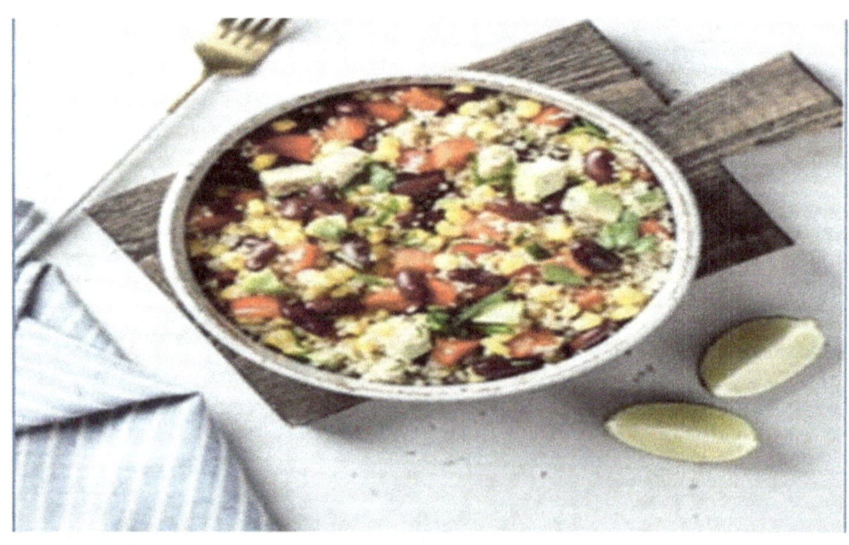

Mediterranean Chickpea and Spinach Stew

A hearty chickpea and spinach stew infused with Mediterranean flavors—ideal for a fulfilling and tasty lunch.

 Cooking/Prep Time: 30 mins 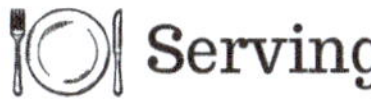 Servings: 2

Ingredients

- One can (15 oz) of rinsed and drained chickpeas
- Two cups of raw spinach
- One 14-oz can of chopped tomatoes
- One sliced onion
- Two minced garlic cloves
- One teaspoon of cumin
- One tsp of paprika
- Half a teaspoon of cilantro
- One tablespoon of olive oil
- Spice to taste

Nutritional Value (Per Serving)

Calories: 320 | Carbs:50g | Protein: 15g | Fats: 8g | Fiber: 14g

Directions

1. Sauté garlic and onions in olive oil in a skillet until they become tender.
2. Stir in diced tomatoes, cumin, paprika, and coriander. Add chickpeas. Allow to simmer for fifteen minutes.
3. Pour in fresh spinach, stir, and allow to wilt.
4. After seasoning, serve warm.

Make Ahead Tips

Make the stew ahead of time and reheat it for a fast midday meal. If necessary, add a little amount of vegetable broth.

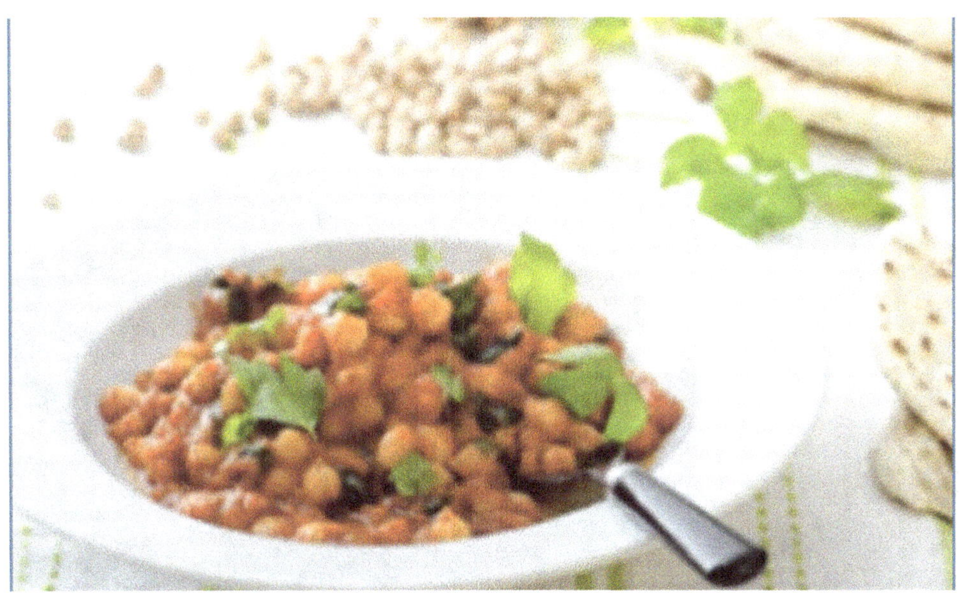

Greek Chicken Souvlaki Wrap

This whole-grain wrap filled with marinated chicken, tzatziki, and vegetables is a popular Mediterranean dish called chicken souvlaki.

 Cooking/Prep Time: 25 mins 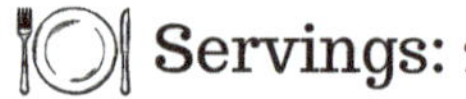 Servings: 2

Ingredients

- One half-pound cut chicken breast and two whole-grain wraps
- Half a cup of cherry tomatoes, 1/2 cucumber cut in half,
- 1/4 cup of red onion finely sliced,
- A quarter cup of crumbled feta cheese
- Tzatziki sauce
- Fresh dill for garnish

Nutritional Value (Per Serving)

Calories: 400 | Carbs:30g | Protein: 30g | Fats: 18g | Fiber: 6g

Directions

1. Give the chicken a 15-minute marinade in a mixture of olive oil, lemon juice, garlic, oregano, salt, and pepper.
2. Cook the chicken thoroughly by grilling or sautéing it.
3. Warm the wraps then, top them with the chicken, feta, tomatoes, cucumbers, red onion, and tzatziki.
4. Add fresh dill as a garnish.

Make Ahead Tips

Marinate the chicken in advance for faster meal.

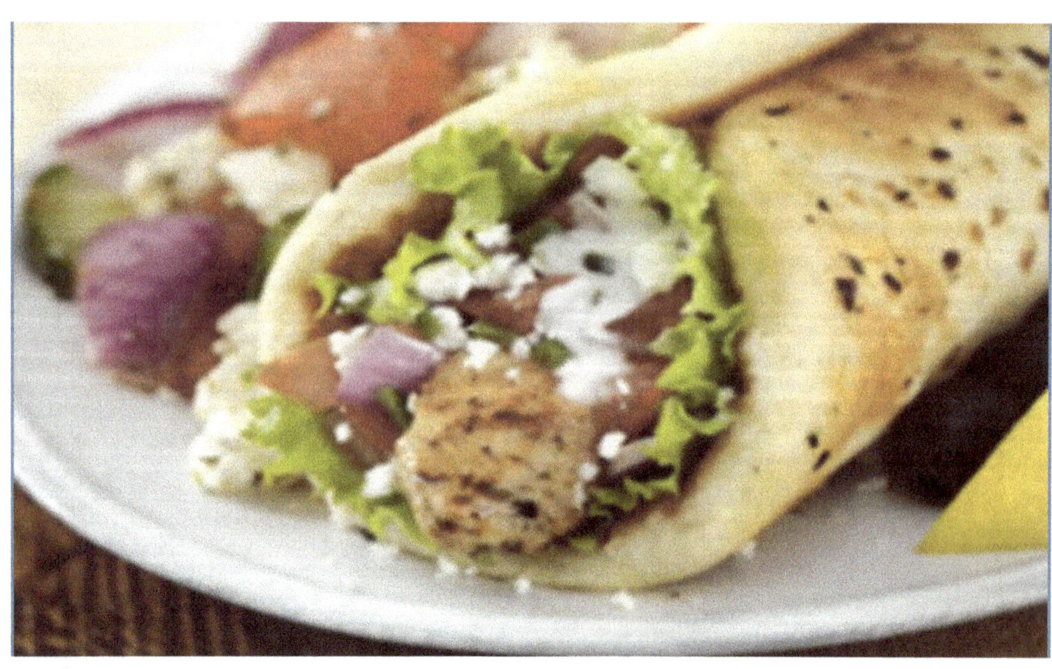

Mediterranean Lentil and Vegetable Stuffed Peppers

A filling and healthy meal prepared from colorful bell peppers filled with a substantial mixture of lentils, vegetables, and Mediterranean spices.

 Cooking/Prep Time: 45 mins 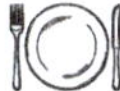 Servings: 2

Ingredients

- Two big bell peppers, seeded and half
- one cup of lentils, cooked
- half a cup of chopped cherry tomatoes
- half a cup of chopped zucchini
- 1/4 cup of coarsely chopped red onion
- 1/4 cup of feta cheese, crumbled
- Two tsp olive oil
- One tsp of dehydrated oregano
- One-half tsp smoked paprika
- Season with pepper and salt

Directions

1. Heat the oven to about 375°F, or 190°C.
2. Combine the cooked lentils, feta, red onion, zucchini, oregano, smoked paprika, olive oil, and salt and pepper in a bowl.
3. Place the lentil mixture into the bell peppers.
4. Bake peppers for 30 to 35 minutes, or until they are soft.

Nutritional Value (Per Serving)

Calories: 380 | Carbs:45g | Protein: 18g | Fats: 14g | Fiber: 12g

Make Ahead Tips

Prepare the lentil stuffing in advance for a quicker lunch.

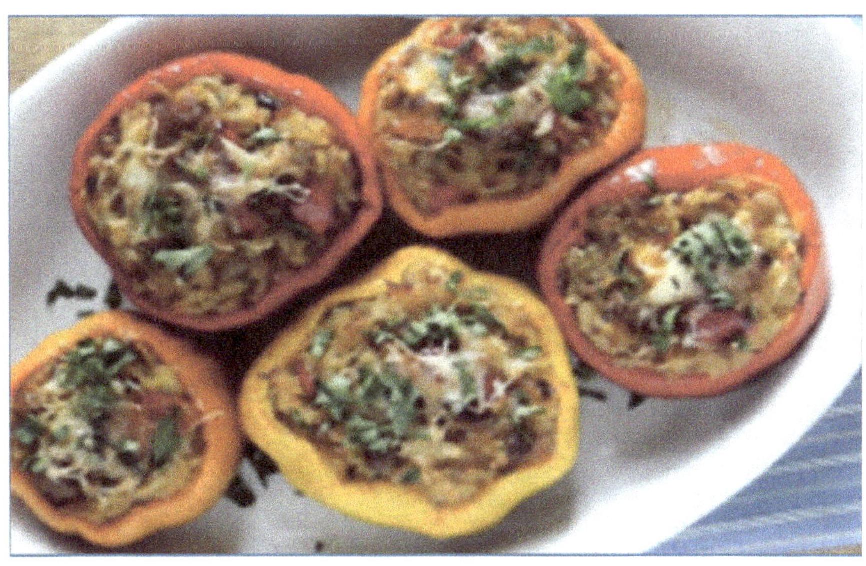

Mediterranean Shrimp and Orzo Salad

A tasty shrimp and orzo salad with vibrant veggies, olives, and a lemony dressing—light yet incredibly flavorful.

 Cooking/Prep Time: 20 mins 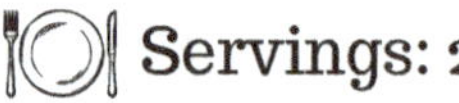 Servings: 2

Ingredients

- Half a pound of shrimp peeled and deveined
- A cup of orzo, cooked
- One cup of cherry tomatoes, halved
- 1/2 cup of cucumber, diced
- A quarter cup of Kalamata olives, sliced
- 1/4 cup of crumbled feta cheese
- Fresh mint leaves for garnish
- Juice of 1 lemon
- Two tablespoons of olive oil
- Spice with salt and pepper.

Directions

1. Cook shrimp thoroughly by sautéing them in olive oil.
2. Toss together cooked orzo, shrimp, cucumber, tomatoes, olives, feta, lemon juice, olive oil, salt, and pepper in a bowl.
3. Add some fresh mint leaves as garnish.

Nutritional Value (Per Serving)

Calories: 420 | Carbs:45g | Protein: 28g | Fats: 16g | Fiber: 4g

Make Ahead Tips

Cook the orzo and sauté the shrimp ahead.

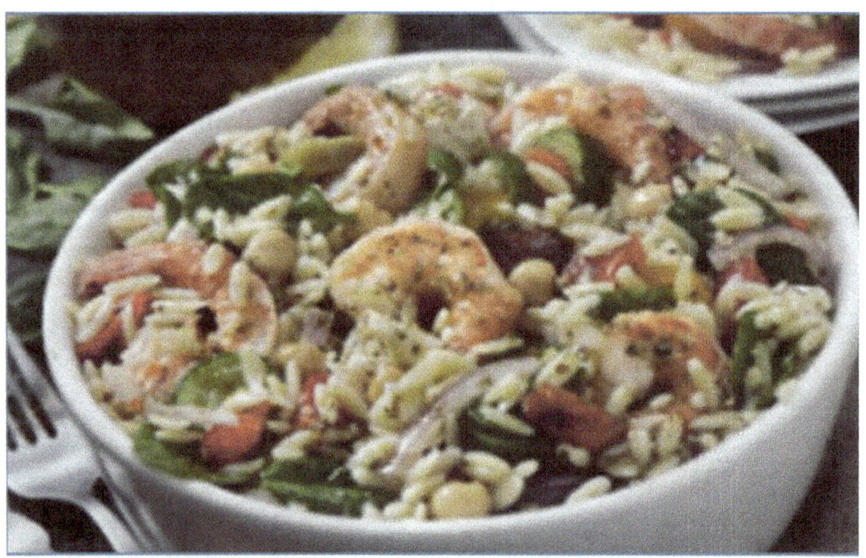

Mediterranean Hummus and Veggie Wrap

A wholesome wrap comprising of hummus, colorful veggies, and a sprinkle of pine nuts—a filling and nutritious Mediterranean lunch.

 Cooking/Prep Time: 15 mins 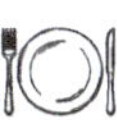 Servings: 2

Ingredients (Hummus)

- One clove of garlic, peeled
- One fifteen-ounce can of chickpeas (garbanzo beans) with no salt
- Three tablespoons of lemon juice
- ü2 tablespoons of olive oil
- A tablespoon of tahini (sesame seed paste)
- A quarter teaspoon of salt
- ¼ teaspoon of white pepper
- A quarter cup of fresh cilantro leaves

ingredients (Wrap)

- Four cups of mixed baby greens
- ½ medium cucumber, sliced
- Half a cup of chopped tomato
- üHalf a cup of thinly sliced red onion
- ¼ cup of crumbled low-fat feta cheese
- Two tablespoons of bottled banana peppers (mildly sliced)
- A tablespoon of balsamic vinegar
- 1 tablespoon of olive oil
- A clove of garlic, minced
- A quarter teaspoon of black pepper
- 2 (8-inch) multi-grain slight tomato-flavored oval wraps

Nutritional Value (Per Serving)

Calories: 340 | Carbs:32g | Protein: 12g | Fats: 18g | Fiber: 10g

Directions

1. To make cilantro hummus, put one peeled garlic clove through the feed tube of a food processor equipped with a steel blade attachment and process until the garlic is finely chopped, while the motor is running. Go over the bowl's sides with a scrape.

2. Garbanzo beans (chickpeas) should be rinsed and drained. Stir in tahini (sesame seed paste), lemon juice, olive oil, garbanzo beans, salt, and white pepper. Process until smooth, scraping down the sides as needed, pausing occasionally. Add the raw cilantro leaves. Once the cilantro is chopped and spread uniformly, pulse a few times. Cool until you use it.

3. mix greens, cucumber, tomato, red onion, feta cheese, and banana peppers in a large bowl to make Mediterranean Wraps. Mix the vinegar, black pepper, garlic, and olive oil in a small bowl. Drizzle the dressing mixture over the combination of greens. Mix by tossing.

4. Distribute around 2 1/2 teaspoons of hummus over each wrap. Garnish with the dressed green combination. Pinch yourself. Present right away.

Make Ahead Tips

Hummus may be created up to three days in advance and refrigerated.

Mediterranean Hummus and Veggie Wrap

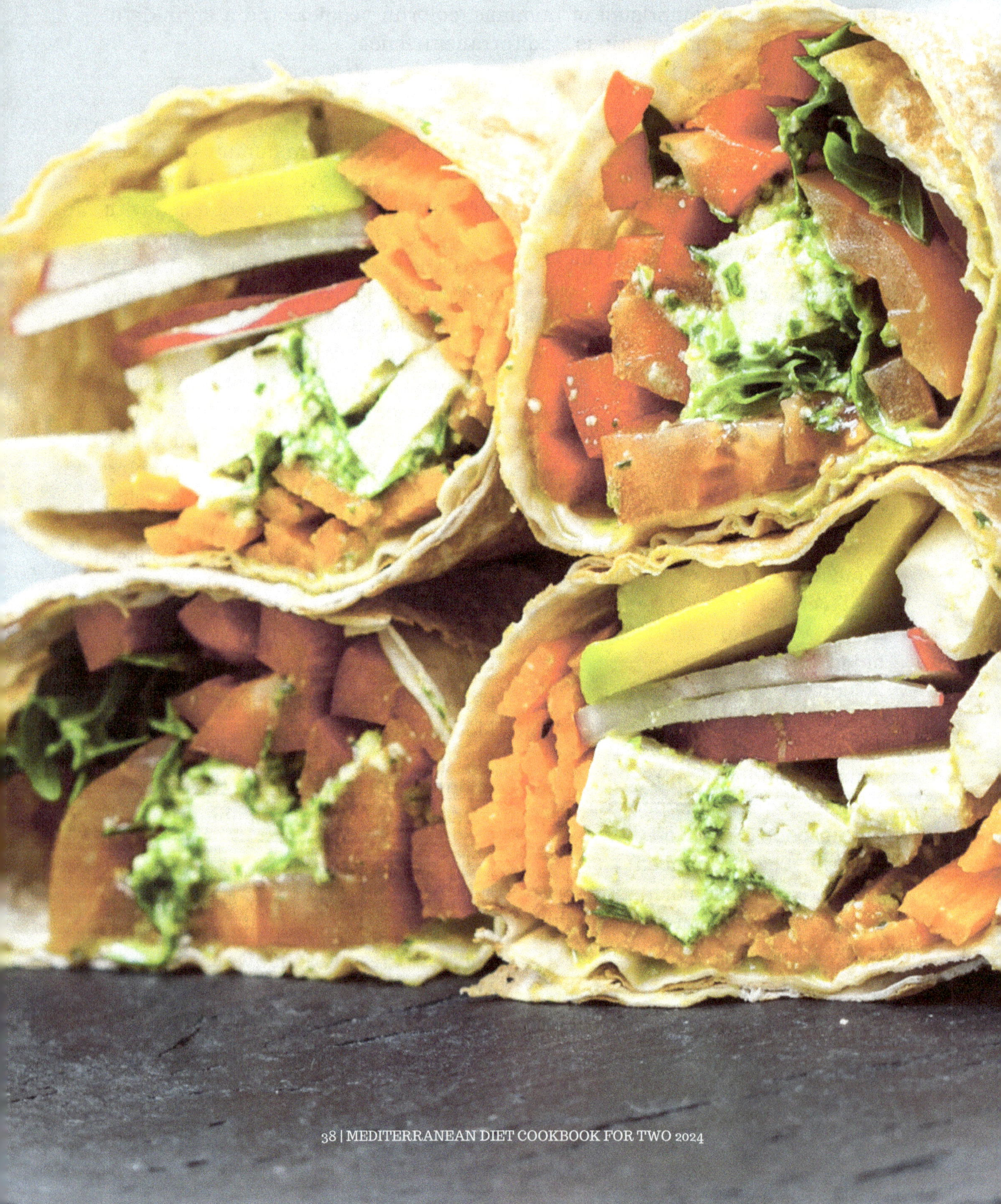

Mediterranean Grilled Vegetable and Quinoa Bowl

A highly nutritious bowl featuring grilled veggies, protein-rich quinoa, and a drizzle of balsamic glaze—a wholesome lunch option.

 Cooking/Prep Time: 30 mins 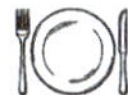 Servings: 2

Ingredients

- One cup of cooked quinoa,
- One sliced zucchini,
- One sliced yellow bell pepper,
- One cup of cherry tomatoes
- 1/2 chopped red onion
- 1/4 cup of feta cheese crumbles
- Balsamic reduction
- For garnish, use fresh basil.

Directions

1. Grill red onion, bell pepper, cherry tomatoes, and zucchini until they start to become a little browned.
2. Transfer cooked quinoa into two bowls.
3. Drizzle some balsamic glaze, feta, and grilled vegetables over top.
4. Add fresh basil as a garnish.

Nutritional Value (Per Serving)

Calories: 380 | Carbs:50g | Protein: 16g | Fats: 12g | Fiber: 8g

Make Ahead Tips

To make preparation time efficient, cook the quinoa and grill the vegetables at the same time.

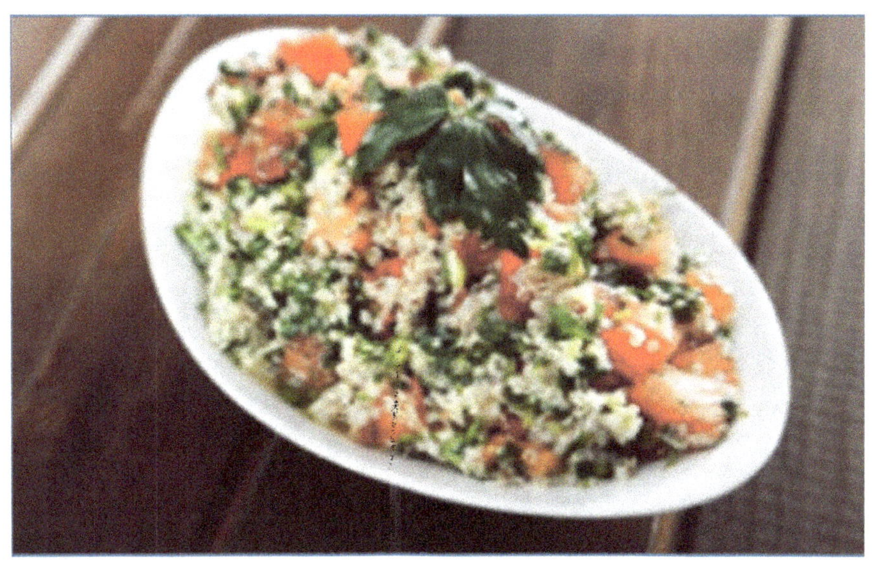

Mediterranean Stuffed Portobello Mushrooms

Hearty Portobello mushrooms stuffed with a mix of quinoa, spinach, and Mediterranean spices—a flavorful andsatisfying lunch.

 Cooking/Prep Time: 40 mins 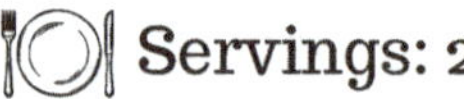 Servings: 2

Ingredients

- Four large Portobello mushroom stems removed
- One cup of quinoa, cooked
- 2 cups of fresh spinach, chopped
- A quarter cup of sun-dried tomatoes, chopped
- 1/4 cup of black olives, sliced
- A quarter cup of crumbled feta cheese
- Two tablespoons of olive oil
- A teaspoon of dried oregano
- Season with pepper and salt

Directions

1. Adjust oven temperature to 375°F or 190°C.
2. Combine cooked quinoa, chopped spinach, sun-dried tomatoes, feta, olives, oregano, olive oil, salt, and pepper in a bowl.
3. Fill each Portobello mushroom with the mixture of quinoa.
4. Bake the mushrooms for 25-30 minutes, or until they are soft.

Nutritional Value (Per Serving)

Calories: 360 | Carbs:45g | Protein: 16g | Fats: 14g | Fiber: 10g

Make Ahead Tips

Prepare the quinoa mixture ahead.

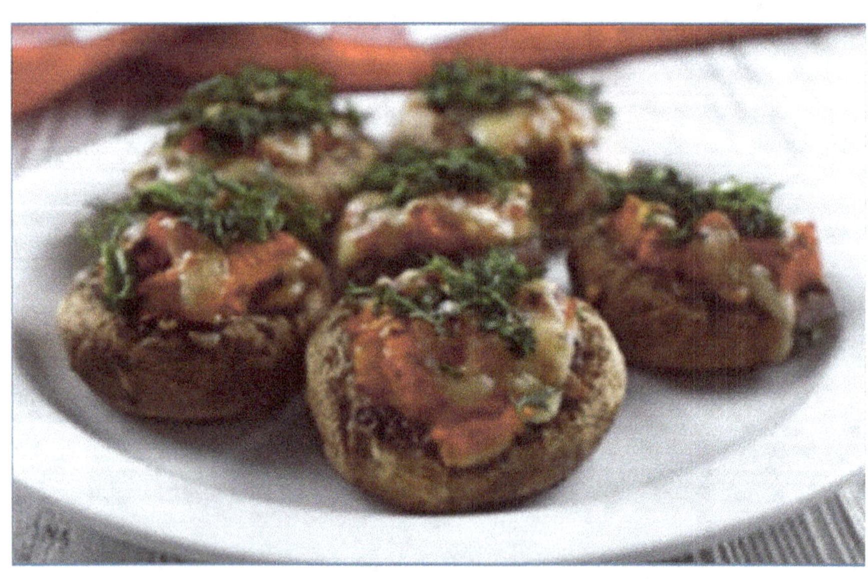

Mediterranean Turkey and Vegetable Skewers

Yummy and tasty skewers featuring turkey, colorful vegetables, and a Mediterranean marinade—perfect for a light and flavorful lunch.

 Cooking/Prep Time: 30 mins 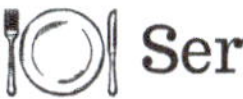 Servings: 2

Ingredients

- Half-pound turkey breast, cut into cubes
- One zucchini, sliced
- One yellow bell pepper, diced
- Half pint of cherry tomatoes
- 1/4 cup of red onion, diced
- Two tablespoons of olive oil
- A teaspoon of dried oregano
- 1 teaspoon of smoked paprika
- Juice of one lime
- Season to taste

Directions

1. Combine the turkey cubes, olive oil, paprika, oregano, lime juice, salt, and pepper in a bowl. Give it fifteen minutes to marinate.
2. Red onion, bell pepper, zucchini, cherry tomatoes, and marinated turkey should all be woven into skewers.
3. Until the turkey is cooked through and the vegetables have a hint of sear, grill or broil the skewers.

Nutritional Value (Per Serving)

Calories: 320 | Carbs:18g | Protein: 30g | Fats: 15g | Fiber: 5g

Make Ahead Tips

Marinate the turkey in advance for enhanced flavor.

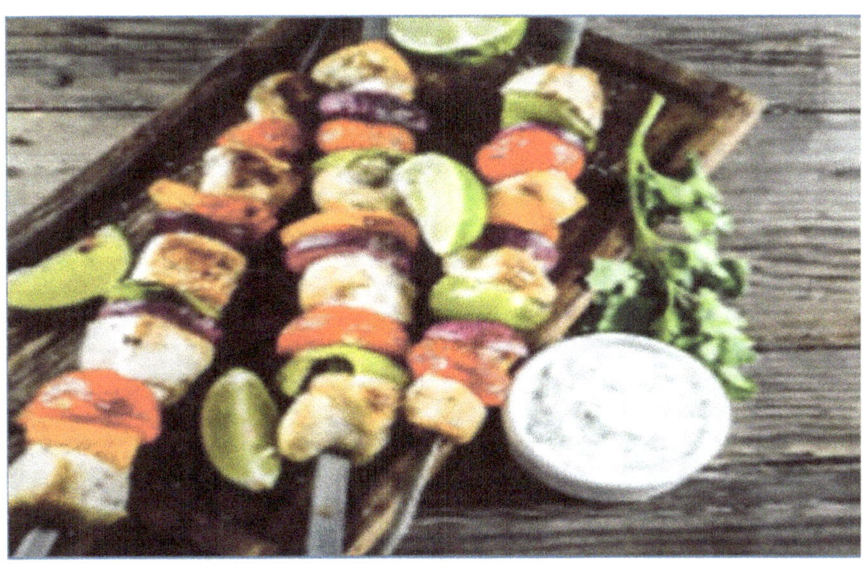

Mediterranean Farro Salad with Roasted Vegetables

A filling and nourishing salad meal consisting of roasted vegetables, nutty farro, and a lemon-oregano vinaigrette.

 Cooking/Prep Time: 45 mins Servings: 2

Ingredients

- A cup of farro, cooked
- 1 zucchini, sliced
- One red bell pepper, sliced
- A cup of cherry tomatoes, halved
- 1/4 cup of red onion, thinly sliced
- Two tablespoons of feta cheese, crumbled
- 2 tablespoons of fresh oregano, chopped
- Two tablespoons of olive oil
- A single lemon's juice
- Seasonings

Directions

1. Roast the bell pepper, cherry tomatoes, and zucchini until they are soft.
2. Toss together cooked farro, feta, red onion, roasted vegetables, oregano, olive oil, lemon juice, salt, and pepper in a bowl.
3. After a little toss, serve.

Nutritional Value (Per Serving)

Calories: 390 | Carbs:50g | Protein: 10g | Fats: 18g | Fiber: 8g

Make Ahead Tips

Cook farro and roast vegetables ahead.

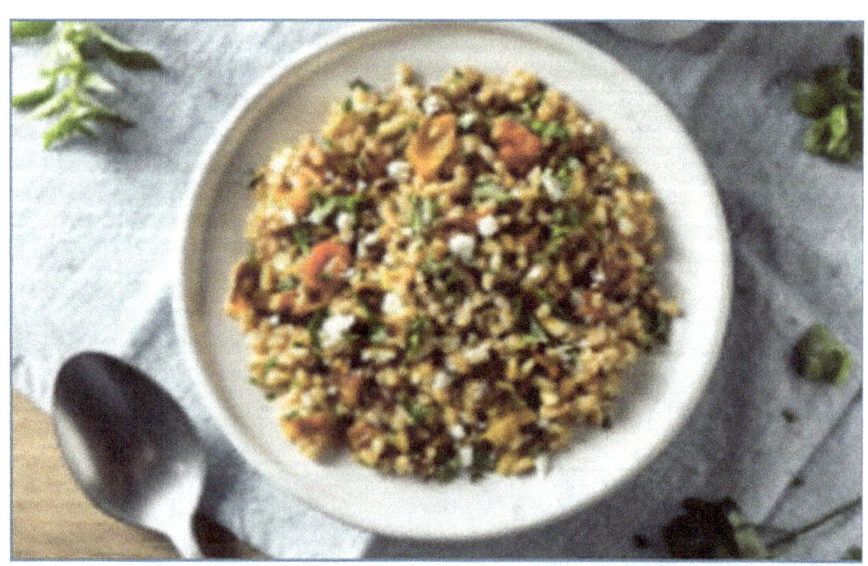

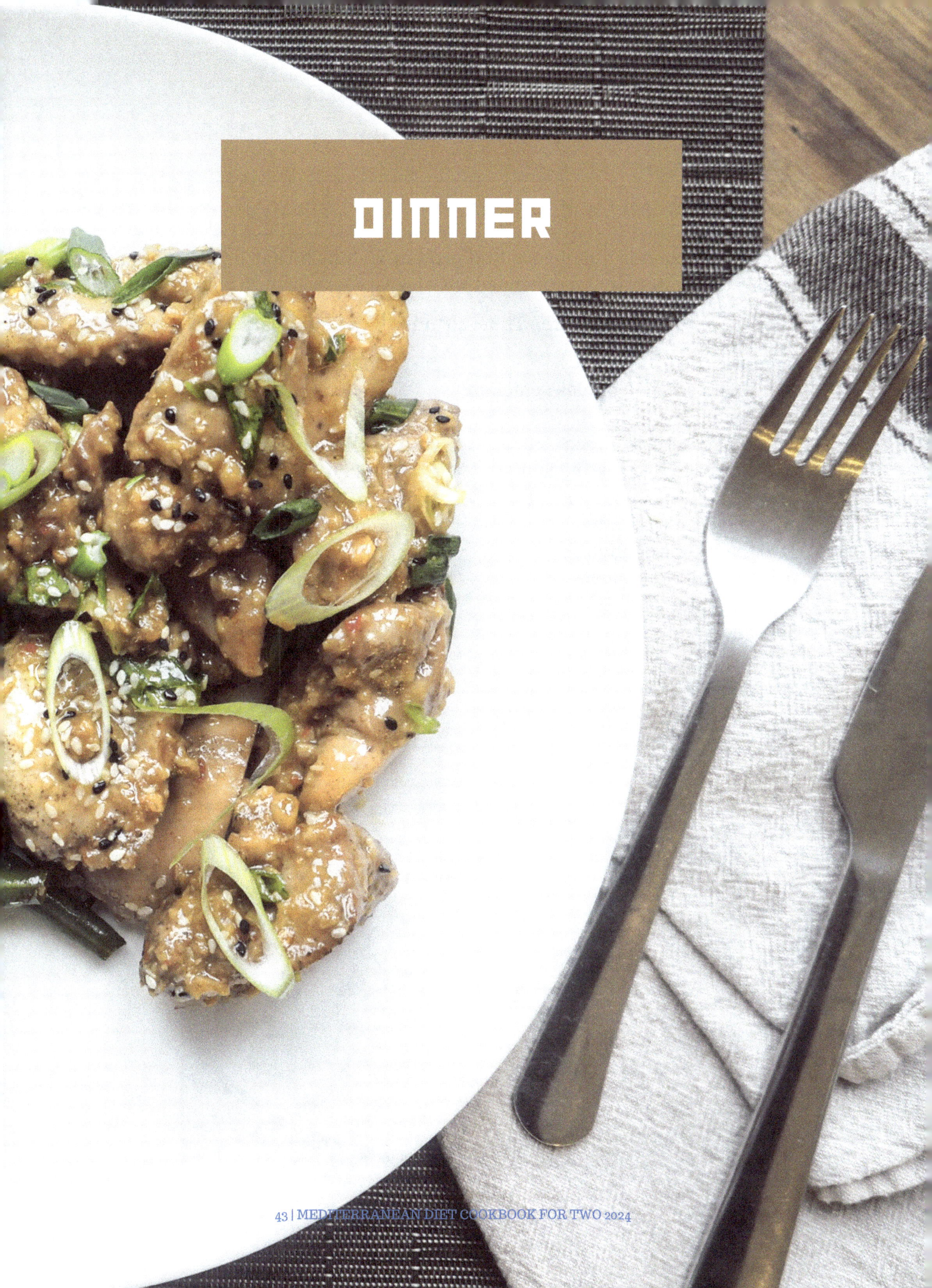

DINNER

Mediterranean Grilled Chicken with Lemon-Herb Quinoa

This grilled chicken is a delicious and protein-rich dish that lets you enjoy the tastes of the Mediterranean combined with a zesty lemon-herb quinoa.

🕐 Cooking/Prep Time: 40 mins 🍽 Servings: 2

Ingredients

- Two skinless and boneless chicken breasts
- One cooked cup of quinoa
- One squeezed and zesting lemon
- Two tablespoons of freshly chopped parsley
- Two teaspoons of olive oil
- two minced garlic cloves
- One tsp of dehydrated oregano
- Season to taste

Directions

1. Give the chicken a 20-minute marinade in a mixture of lemon juice, zest, garlic, oregano, salt, and pepper.
2. Chicken should be cooked through on the grill.
3. Add olive oil, parsley, salt, and pepper to cooked quinoa.
4. Over a layer of lemon-herb quinoa, serve grilled chicken.

Nutritional Value (Per Serving)

Calories: 420 | Carbs: 30g | Protein: 35g | Fats: 18g | Fiber: 4g

Make Ahead Tips

To enhance the flavor of the chicken, marinate it in advance.

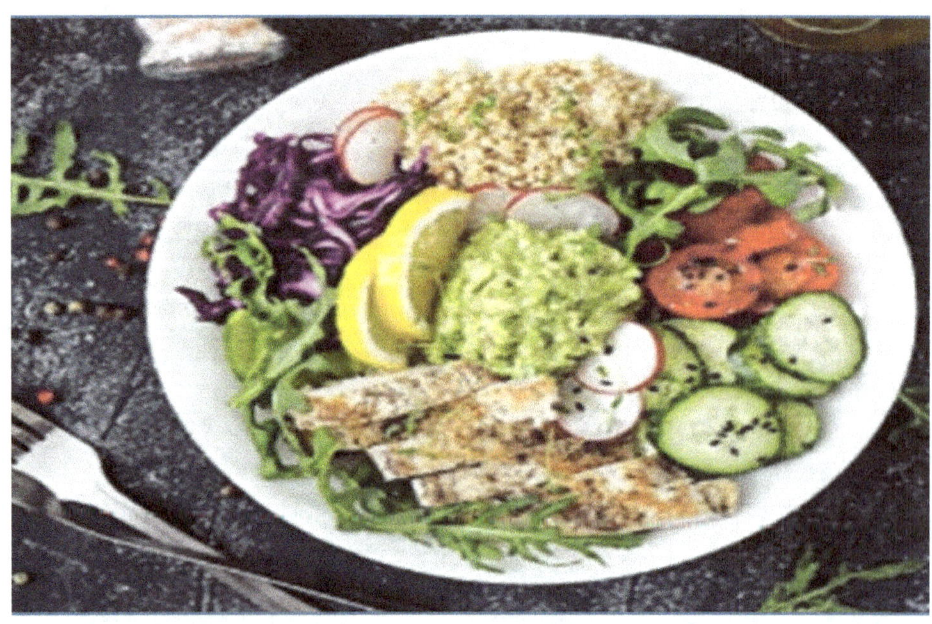

Mediterranean Baked Salmon with Roasted Vegetables

This tasty and heart-healthy baked salmon, topped with a mix of roasted veggies, will elevate your dinner.

 Cooking/Prep Time: 35 mins 🍽 Servings: 2

Ingredients

- Two fillets of salmon
- One sliced zucchini
- One sliced red bell pepper
- Half a cup of cherry tomatoes
- two tsp of capers
- Two tsp olive oil
- A single tsp of dried thyme
- Juice of 1 lemon
- Season to taste

Nutritional Value (Per Serving)

Calories: 380 | Carbs: 15g | Protein: 30g | Fats: 22g | Fiber: 4g

Directions

1. Put the oven on to 375°F, or 190°C.
2. Arrange the salmon on a baking sheet and top with the veggies, lemon juice, olive oil, capers, thyme, salt, and pepper.
3. Bake the veggies until they are soft and the salmon is cooked through.

Make Ahead Tips

Prepare the vegetable medley in ahead for faster meal.

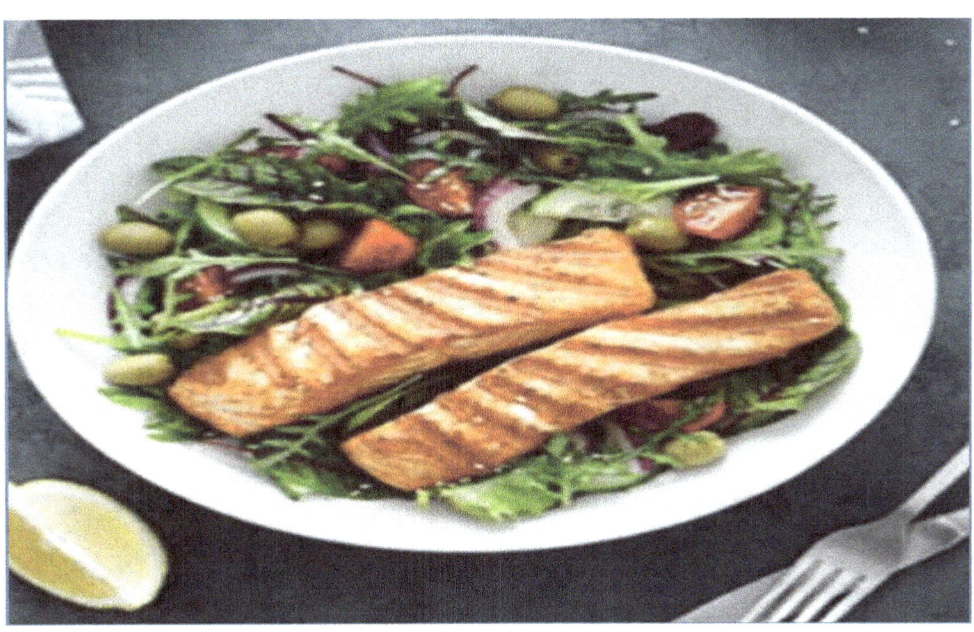

Skillet Lemon Chicken and potatoes with Kale

A one-pot marvel that blends tender chicken, filling potatoes, and kale that is high in nutrients, all enhanced by the bright, zesty flavor of lemon.

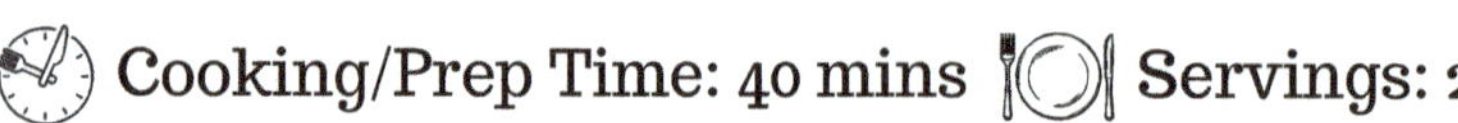 Cooking/Prep Time: 40 mins Servings: 2

Ingredients

- Two skin-on, bone-in chicken thighs
- One cup of halved baby potatoes
- Two cups chopped kale (stems removed)
- One thinly sliced lemon
- Three minced garlic cloves
- Two tsp olive oil
- A single tsp of dried thyme
- One tsp of dehydrated rosemary
- Salt and pepper

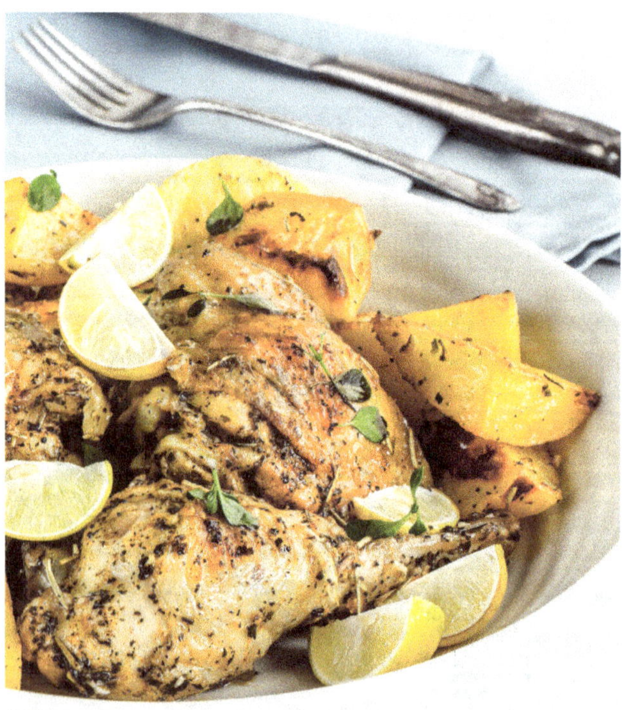

Directions

1. Adjust oven temperature to 400°F or 200°C.
2. Add a little salt, pepper, thyme, and rosemary to the chicken thighs.
3. Heat the olive oil in a skillet that is oven-safe to medium-high heat. Chicken thighs should be seared until all sides are golden brown.
4. Potato halves should be added to the pan and arranged around the chicken.
5. Divide the chopped kale among the potatoes and chicken. Distribute the minced garlic equally.
6. Arrange the lemon slices over the chicken. Over the veggies, drizzle a little more olive oil.
7. After placing the pan in the preheated oven, bake it for 25 to 30 minutes, or until the potatoes are soft and the chicken achieves an internal temperature of 165°F (74°C).
8. For a golden finish, broil for a further three to five minutes

Make Ahead Tips

Pre-cut potatoes and kale to streamline the preparation process.

Nutritional Value (Per Serving)

Calories: 380 | Carbs: 20g | Protein: 25g | Fats: 22g | Fiber: 5g

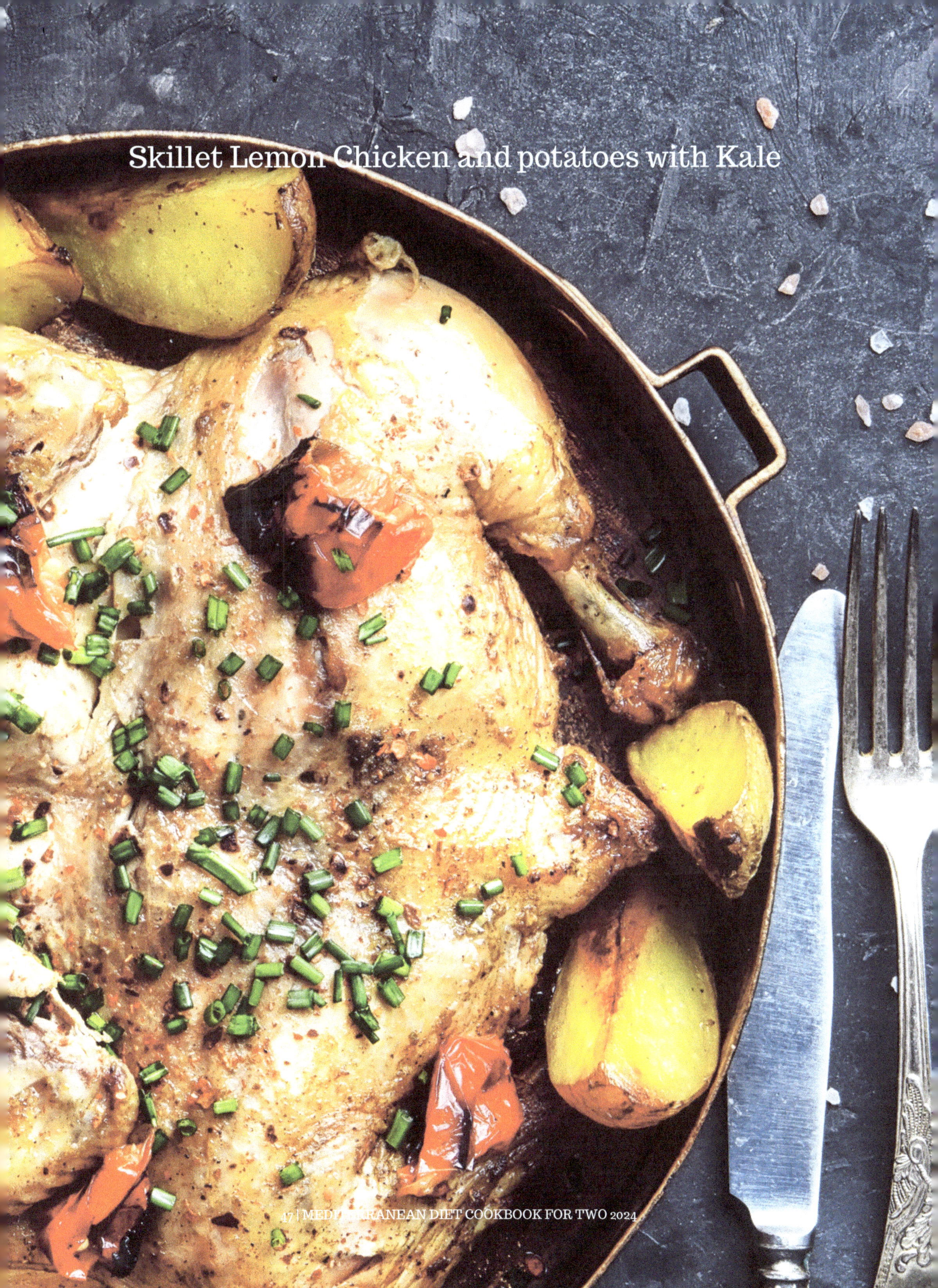

Skillet Lemon Chicken and potatoes with Kale

Mediterranean Lentil Soup with Spinach

Warm up your evening with this hearty lentil soup, packed with protein and vibrant spinach—a delighful and nutrient-packed dinner.

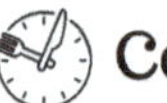 Cooking/Prep Time: 45 mins 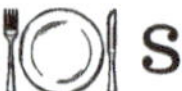 Servings: 2

Ingredients

- One cup of dry green lentils, washed
- Four cups of vegetable broth/water
- One onion, chopped;
- Two carrots
- Two celery stalks; chopped;
- Three minced garlic cloves
- Two cups of raw spinach
- One teaspoon each of cumin and smoked paprika
- Two tsp of olive oil
- Season taste

Nutritional Value (Per Serving)

Calories: 340 | Carbs: 50g | Protein: 18g | Fats: 8g | Fiber: 18g

Directions

1. Add the garlic, celery, carrots, and onions to a saucepan containing olive oil and sauté until softened.
2. Stir in lentils, smoked paprika, cumin, and vegetable broth. Season with salt and pepper. Lentils should be cooked until soft.
3. Lastly, stir in the fresh spinach and allow it to simmer until moderately soft.
4. Serve warm!

Cooking Tips

- Prepare the soup in larger batches for freezing.
- Soak lentils for ten to fifteen minutes to expedite the cooking process.
- Next, add to the pan after draining.

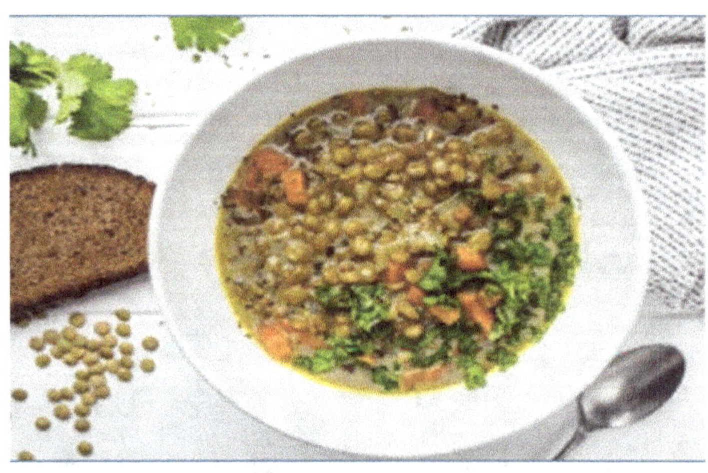

Mediterranean Shrimp Pasta with Tomato-Basil Sauce

Enjoy a delicious supper of fast and flavorful Mediterranean shrimp pasta with a tomato-basil sauce.

 Cooking/Prep Time: 15 mins   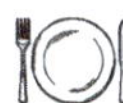 Servings: 2

Ingredients

- Eight oz of whole-grain spaghetti, cooked
- Twelve large shrimp, peeled and deveined
- A cup of cherry tomatoes, halved
- 1/4 cup of fresh basil, chopped
- Two cloves garlic, minced
- 2 tablespoons of olive oil
- Juice of 1 lemon
- Red pepper flakes (optional)
- Salt and pepper as desired

Directions

1. Garlic, cherry tomatoes, and shrimp should be sautéed in olive oil until the shrimp are done.
2. Mix the cooked spaghetti with the combination of shrimp.
3. Incorporate the lemon juice, red pepper flakes, fresh basil, salt, and pepper. Allow it to simmer for 2 minutes, then enjoy!

Nutritional Value (Per Serving)

Calories: 450 | Carbs: 60g | Protein: 25g | Fats: 15g | Fiber: 8g

Make Ahead Tips

Cook the pasta ahead of time for a quicker preparation.

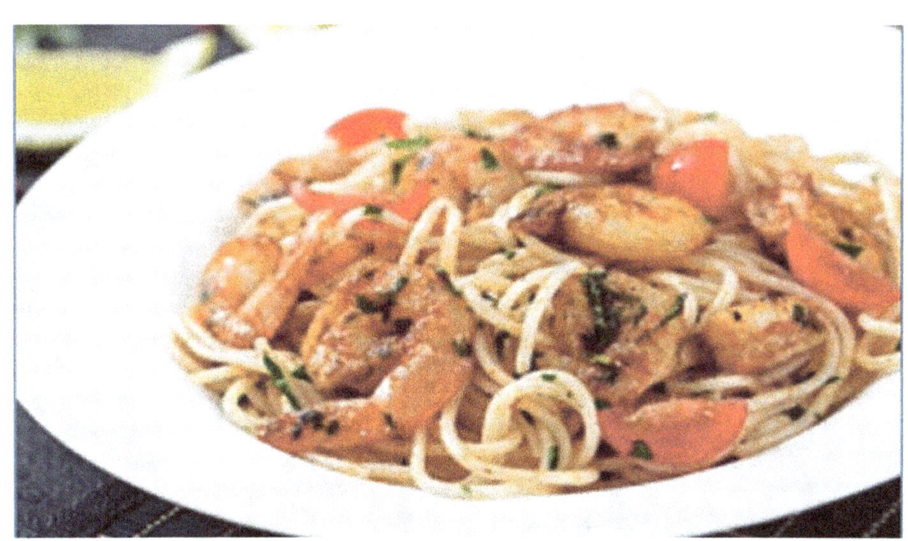

Mediterranean Chickpea Salad with Lemon-Tahini Dressing

Enjoy a refreshing and protein-packed dinner with this Mediterranean chickpea salad, drizzled with a zesty lemon-tahini dressing.

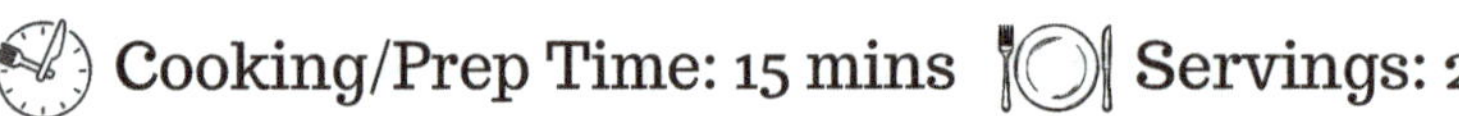 Cooking/Prep Time: 15 mins   Servings: 2

Ingredients

- A can of chickpeas, drained and rinsed
- One cucumber, diced
- A cup of cherry tomatoes, halved
- 1/4 cup of red onion, finely chopped
- A quarter cup of Kalamata olives, sliced
- 1/4 cup of feta cheese, crumbled
- Two tablespoons of olive oil
- 2 tablespoons of lemon juice
- A tablespoon of tahini
- 1 teaspoon of dried oregano
- Salt and pepper

Directions

1. Chickpeas, cucumber, cherry tomatoes, red onion, olives, and feta should all be combined in a bowl.
2. For the dressing, whisk together olive oil, lemon juice, tahini, oregano, salt, and pepper.
3. Mix the lemon-tahini dressing into the salad. Serve!

Make Ahead Tips

Prepare the dressing separately and add just before serving.

Nutritional Value (Per Serving)

Calories: 380 | Carbs: 40g | Protein: 16g | Fats: 18g | Fiber: 10g

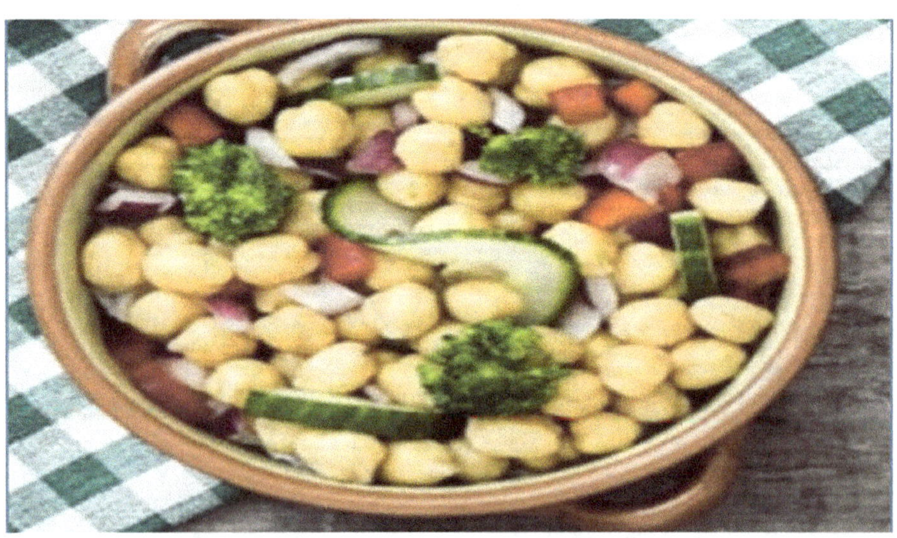

Mediterranean Stuffed Bell Pepper with Ground Turkey

Savor a delicious meal by stuffing bell peppers with a flavorful blend of ground turkey and Mediterranean spices.

 Cooking/Prep Time: 55 mins  Servings: 2

Ingredients

- Two large bell peppers, halved and seeds removed
- Half a pound of ground turkey
- A cup of cooked quinoa
- 1/2 cup of cherry tomatoes, diced
- A quarter cup of feta cheese, crumbled
- 1/4 cup of black olives, sliced
- One teaspoon of dried oregano
- A teaspoon of ground cumin
- Two tablespoons of olive oil
- Season to taste

Nutritional Value (Per Serving)

Calories: 420 | Carbs: 35g | Protein: 28g | Fats: 20g | Fiber: 7g

Directions

1. Set oven temperature to 375°F or 190°C.
2. Combine oregano, cumin, salt, and pepper with ground turkey and brown it in olive oil.
3. Combine the turkey mixture with the cooked quinoa, feta, cherry tomatoes, and black olives.
4. Stuff with bell peppers and bake till the peppers are soft.

Make Ahead Tips

Prepare the turkey and quinoa mixture in ahead.

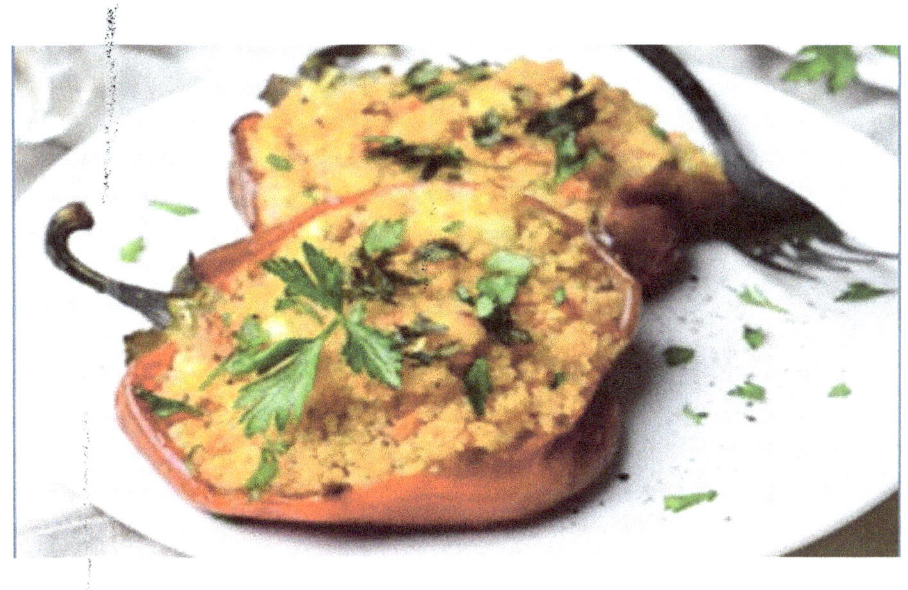

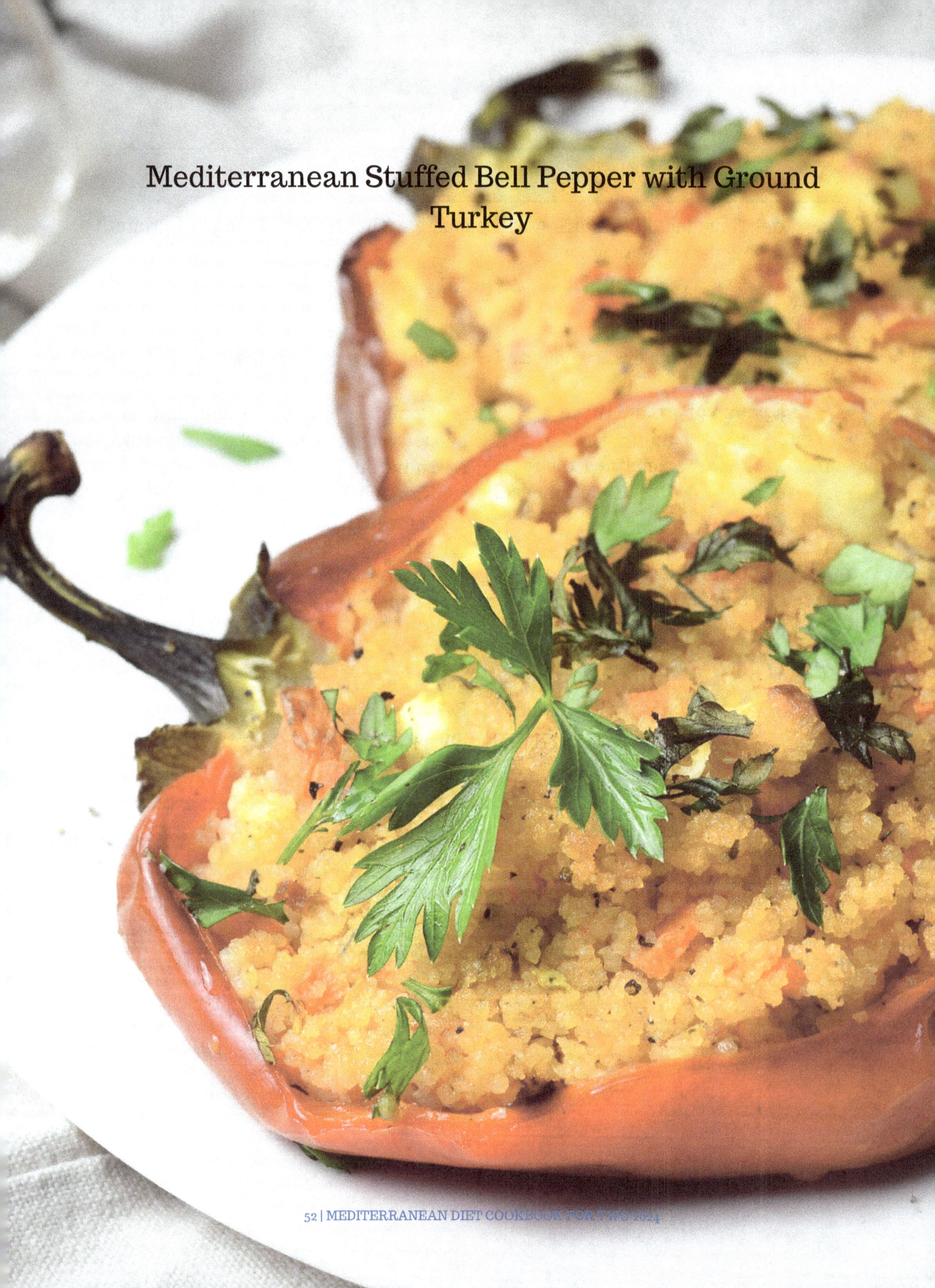

Mediterranean Stuffed Bell Pepper with Ground Turkey

Mediterranean Veggie Pita Wrap with Tzatziki

Enjoy a tasty and light Mediterranean veggie pita at the end of the day, topped with creamy tzatziki sauce and crisp veggies.

 Cooking/Prep Time: 20 mins 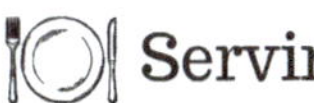 Servings: 2

Ingredients

- Two (2) whole-grain pita bread rounds
- A cup of cherry tomatoes, halved
- One cucumber, sliced
- 1/2 a cup of red bell pepper, sliced
- 1/4 cup of red onion, thinly sliced
- A quarter cup of feta cheese, crumbled
- 1/4 cup of Kalamata olives, sliced
- Half a cup of Greek yogurt
- One tablespoon of fresh dill, chopped
- A tablespoon of lemon juice
- Salt and pepper as desired

Directions

1. Combine cherry tomatoes, cucumber, red onion, red bell pepper, feta, and olives in a bowl.
2. To make the tzatziki sauce, mix Greek yogurt, dill, lemon juice, salt, and pepper in another bowl.
3. Fill warmed pita bread with vegetable mixture. Top with a drizzle of tzatziki sauce.

Make Ahead Tips

Prepare the tzatziki sauce separately and add it right before serving.

Nutritional Value (Per Serving)

Calories: 320 | Carbs: 40g | Protein: 12g | Fats: 12g | Fiber: 6g

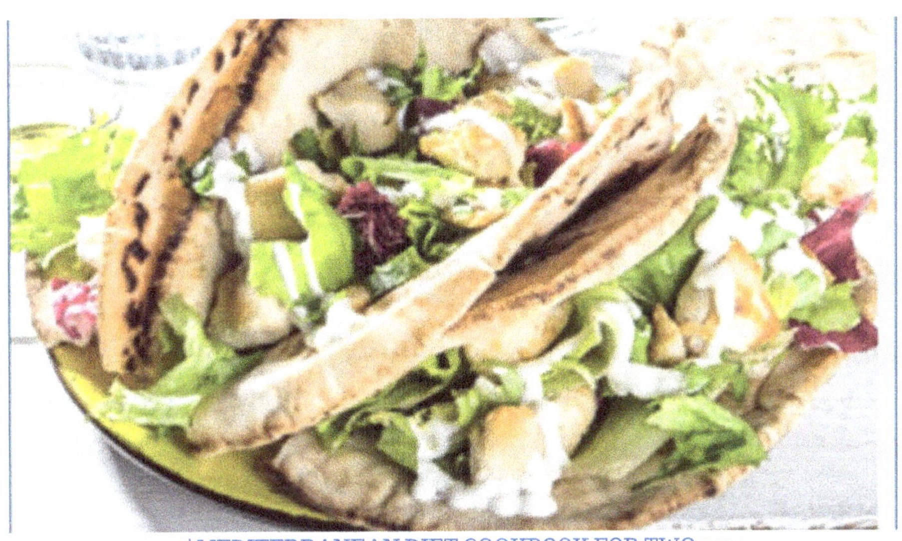

Mediterranean Eggplant and Chickpea Bake

This grilled chicken is a delicious and protein-rich dish that lets you enjoy the tastes of the Mediterranean combined with a zesty lemon-herb quinoa.

 Cooking/Prep Time: 45 mins 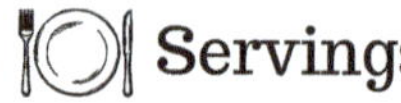 Servings: 2

Ingredients

- One large eggplant, sliced
- A can of chickpeas, drained and rinsed
- One cup of cherry tomatoes, halved
- 1/4 cup of red onion, thinly sliced
- Two cloves of garlic, minced
- 2 tablespoons of olive oil
- A teaspoon of dried thyme
- One teaspoon of ground cumin
- Salt and pepper

Directions

1. Set oven temperature to 375°F, or 190°C.
2. In a pan, combine garlic, red onion, thyme, cumin, salt and pepper, eggplant, chickpeas, cherry tomatoes, and red onion in olive oil.
3. Bake until the chickpeas are crunchy and the veggies are soft.

Nutritional Value (Per Serving)

Calories: 380 | Carbs: 45g | Protein: 15g | Fats: 18g | Fiber: 12g

Make Ahead Tips

Prepare the vegetable mixture in advance.

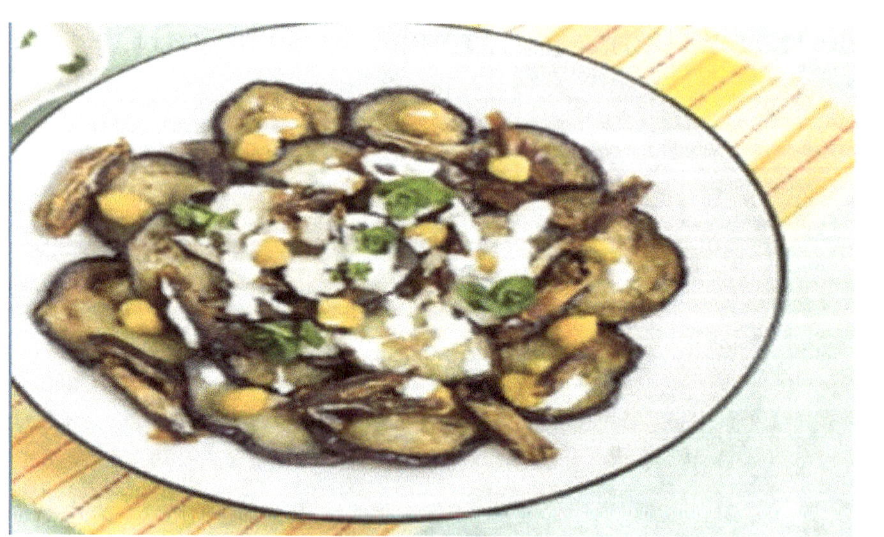

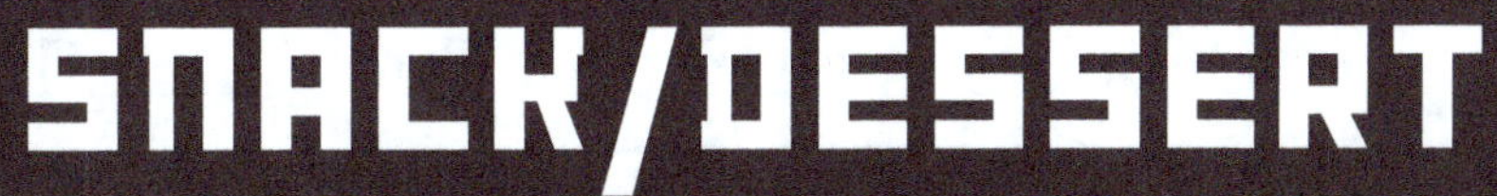
SNACK/DESSERT

SNACKS/DESSERTS

Cranberry-Almond Energy Balls

These bite-sized sweets are loaded with components that promote energy, making them an ideal fast and healthy snack.

 Cooking/Prep Time: 15 mins 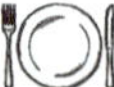 Servings: 2 Yield: 10 Balls

Ingredients

- A cup of rolled oats
- 1/2 cup of almond butter
- A quarter cup of honey
- 1/4 cup of dried cranberries
- A quarter cup of almonds, chopped
- A teaspoon of vanilla extract
- Pinch of salt

Nutritional Value (Per Serving)

Calories: 150 | Carbs: 18g | Protein: 4g | Fats: 8g | Fiber: 3g

Directions

1. Blend together rolled oats, almond butter, honey, sliced almonds, dried cranberries, vanilla essence, and a little amount of salt in a food processor.
2. keep pulsing the ingredients until a sticky dough is achieved (40 to 60 seconds)
3. Form the dough into little balls using wet hands, then arrange them on a tray covered with paper.
4. Chill for a minimum of half an hour before serving.
5. Make Ahead/Cooking Tips:
6. Make a batch and store in an airtight container for a quick grab-and-go snack.

Note:

Due to cross-contamination with wheat and barley, those with celiac disease or gluten sensitivity should only consume "gluten-free" oats.

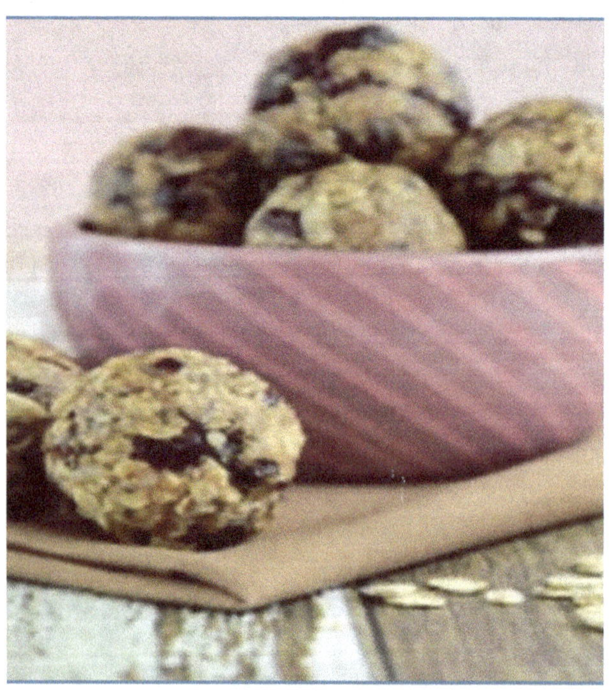

Cottage Cheese with Raspberry Honey

Savor the simplicity of Raspberry Honey with Cottage Cheese, a delicious combination of tart and sweet honey infused with raspberries.

 Cooking/Prep Time: 5 mins 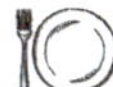 Servings: 2

Ingredients

- A cup of cottage cheese
- 1/4 cup of fresh raspberries
- Two tablespoons of honey

Nutritional Value (Per Serving)

Calories: 220 | Carbs: 24g | Protein: 12g | Fats: 9g | Fiber: 2g

Directions

1.   Transfer cottage cheese into a dishing bowl.
2.   Drizzle some fresh raspberries over it.
3.   Pour a good amount of honey over the raspberries and cottage cheese. Savor!

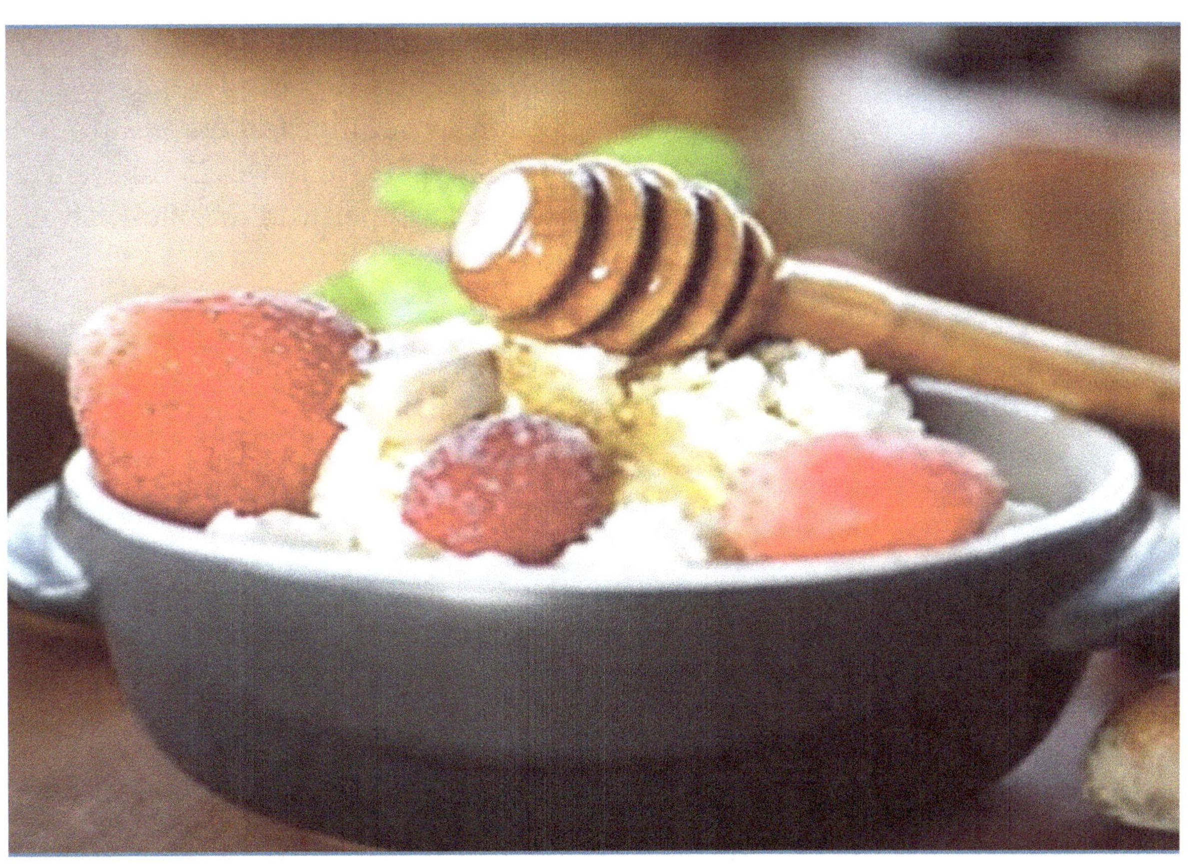

Cauliflower Hummus

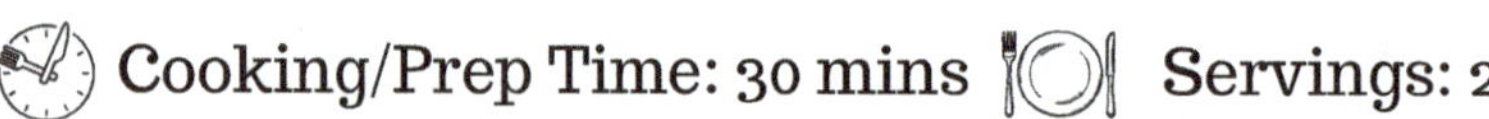

This creamy concoction of tahini, cauliflower, and Mediterranean spices will satisfy your hummus cravings without making you feel guilty.

🕐 Cooking/Prep Time: 30 mins 🍽 Servings: 2

Ingredients

- 3 cups cauliflower florets (about half a pound)
- One tablespoon extra-virgin olive oil, plus more for garnish
- 1 medium garlic clove, roughly chopped
- ¼ cup of tahini
- Zest of 1 lemon
- One tablespoon of lemon juice
- Quarter teaspoon of kosher salt
- A quarter teaspoon of ground cumin
- ¼ teaspoon of crushed red pepper
- 1 tablespoon of water
- Chopped red bell pepper for garnish

Nutritional Value (Per Serving)

Calories: 180 | Carbs: 10g | Protein: 12g | Fats: 15g | Fiber: 4g

Equipment

A parchment paper or silicone baking mat

Directions

1. Line a baking sheet with silicone mats or parchment paper on it and turn on the oven to 400°F. In a big bowl, mix the cauliflower with oil. Then place on the prepared baking sheet by arranging in one layer. Roast for 20 to 25 minutes, or until soft and beginning to brown. Leave it to cool down to room temperature.

2. In a food processor, combine the cauliflower, garlic, tahini, lemon zest, lemon juice, salt, cumin, crushed red pepper, and water. Blend until well incorporated, stopping occasionally to scrape down the bowl's edges. If you want a looser dip, add more water.

3. Move to a bowl. If desired, add chopped pepper and drizzle with more olive oil.

To Make Ahead

Roast cauliflower as explained above and refrigerate in an airtight container for up to 2 days.

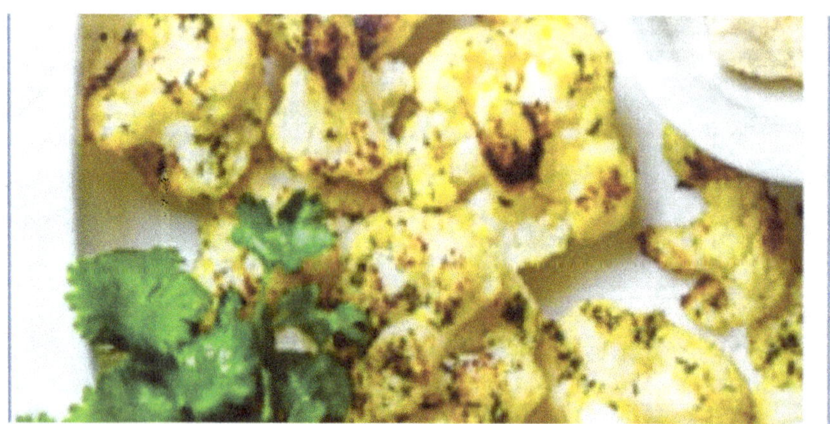

Pretzels with Dark Chocolate & Peanut Butter

A delicious mixture of salty pretzels, rich dark chocolate, and creamy peanut butter that satisfies sweet and savory cravings.

 Cooking/Prep Time: 15 mins 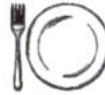 Servings: 2

Ingredients

- One cup of pretzels
- 1/2 cup of dark chocolate, melted
- A quarter cup of peanut butter melted.

Nutritional Value (Per Serving)

Calories: 250 | Carbs: 30g | Protein: 6g | Fats: 12g | Fiber: 2g

Directions

1. Coat the pretzels halfway with melted dark chocolate.

2. Transfer to a tray lined with paper, and allow the chocolate to solidify.

3. Spread melted peanut butter over the pretzels that have been coated in chocolate. Enjoy!

Make Ahead Tips

Prepare a batch and store it in a cool place for an indulgent snack.

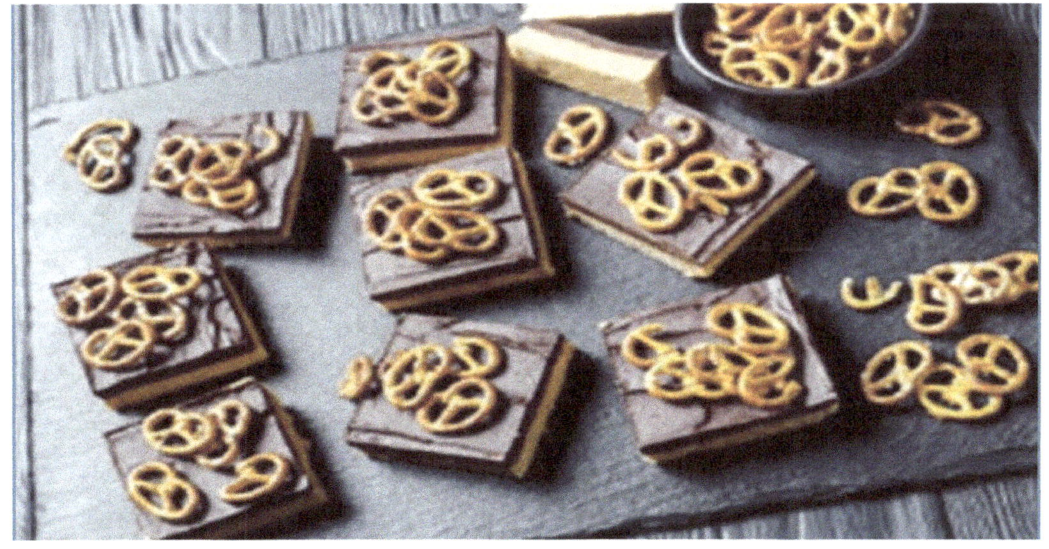

Pineapple Nice Cream

A dairy-free and naturally sweetened frozen treat that captures the essence of the tropics.

🕐 Cooking/Prep Time: 10 mins 🍽 Servings: 2

Ingredients

- Two cups of frozen pineapple chunks
- Half a cup of coconut milk
- 1 tablespoon of honey
- A teaspoon of vanilla extract

Directions

1. Blend together frozen pineapple chunks, honey, coconut milk, and vanilla essence using a blender.
2. Pulse till creamy and smooth.
3. Serve right away.

Nutritional Value (Per Serving)

Calories: 180 | Carbs: 45g | Protein: 2g | Fats: 1g | Fiber: 5g

To Make Ahead

Freeze individual portions for an easy and refreshing dessert.

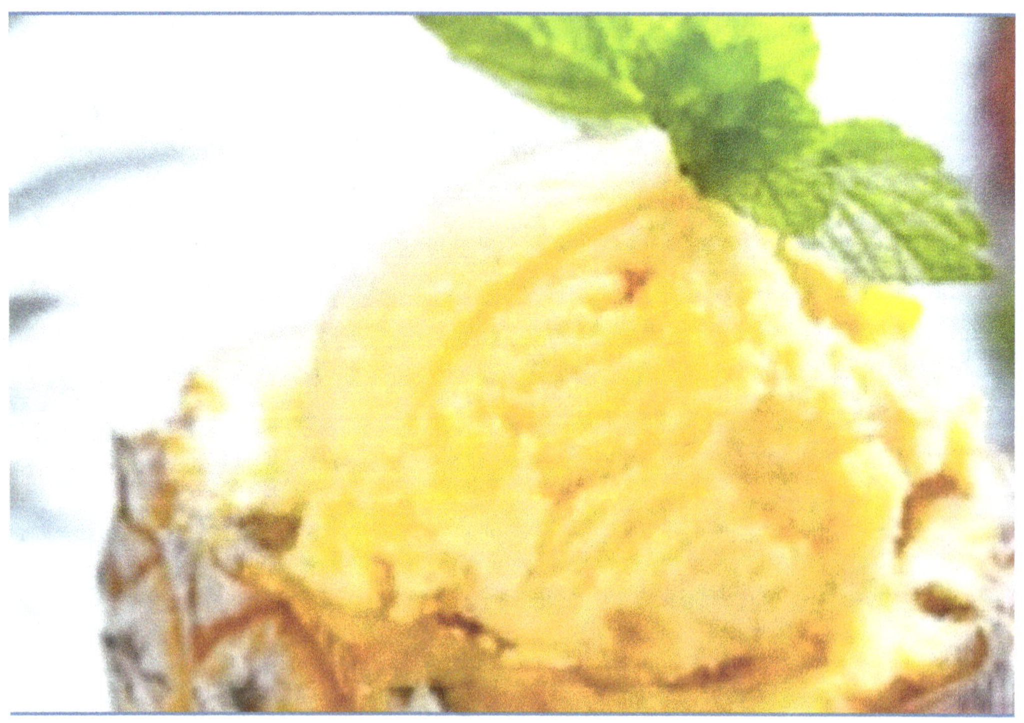

No-Sugar-Added Mini Apple Pies

A healthier twist on a classic dessert, featuring the natural sweetness of apples without any added sugars.

 Cooking/Prep Time: 30 mins 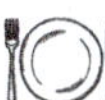 Servings: 2

Ingredients

- Two apples, peeled and diced
- 1 teaspoon of cinnamon
- Half a teaspoon of nutmeg
- 1 tablespoon of lemon juice
- A cup of almond flour
- Two tablespoons of coconut oil, melted
- 1 teaspoon of vanilla extract

Nutritional Value (Per Serving)

Calories: 240 | Carbs: 20g | Protein: 6g | Fats: 16g | Fiber: 6g

Directions

1. Set the oven's temperature to 175°C/350°F.
2. Combine already diced apples with lemon juice, nutmeg, and cinnamon in a basin.
3. To make a crumbly dough, mix almond flour, melted coconut oil, and vanilla essence in a separate basin.
4. Place some of the dough into the tiny pie molds to form the crust.
5. Spoon the spiced apples into each crust.
6. Bake the crust for 20 minutes, or until it becomes brown.

Tips

Prepare the apple filling and almond flour dough in ahead for easy snacking.

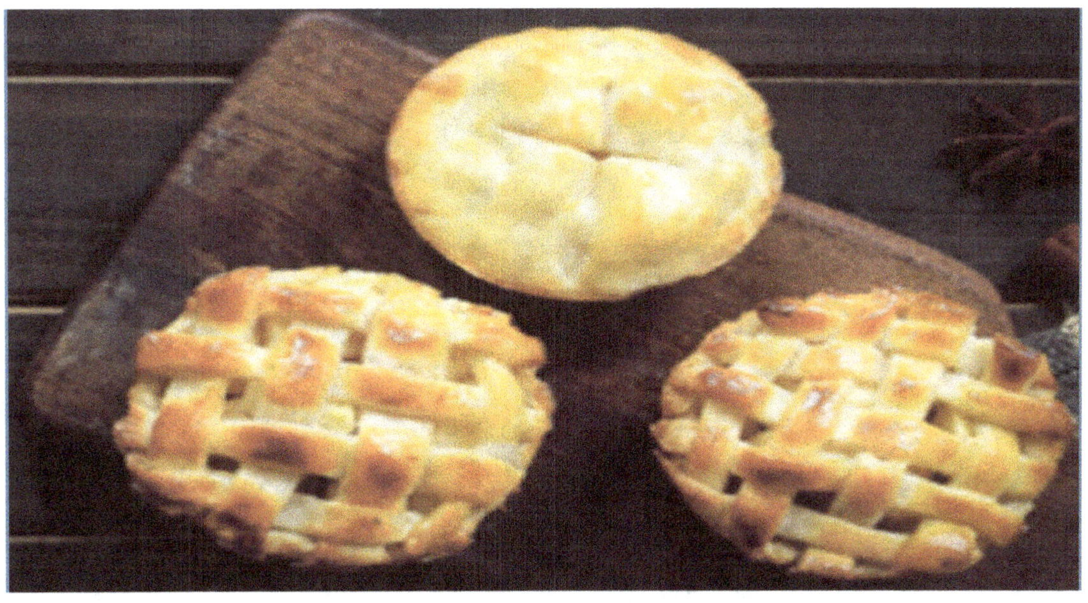

SOUPS

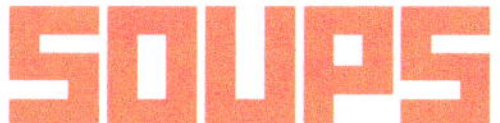

SOUPS

Vegan Cabbage Soup

This Vegan Cabbage Soup—is a hearty blend of vegetables, beans, and cabbage. It is not only flavorful but also an excellent source of plant-based nutrition.

 Cooking/Prep Time: 30 mins 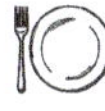 Servings: 2

Ingredients

- One tablespoon of olive oil
- 1 onion, diced
- Two carrots, sliced
- Two celery stalks, chopped
- 3 garlic cloves, minced
- Four cups of vegetable broth
- A can (15 oz) of diced tomatoes
- One small cabbage, shredded
- A can (15 oz) of cannellini beans, well-rinsed and drained
- A teaspoon of thyme
- Season to taste

Directions

1. Warm up the olive oil in a big saucepan over medium heat. Add the garlic, celery, carrots, and onion. Sauté the veggies till they get soft.
2. Add the chopped tomatoes and veggie broth. Heat through to a simmer.
3. Add the cannellini beans, thyme, salt, pepper, and chopped cabbage. Simmer for fifteen more minutes.
4. Before serving, taste and adjust the seasoning.

Nutritional Value (Per Serving)

Calories: 250 | Carbs: 45g | Protein: 10g | Fats: 5g | Fiber: 12g

Make Ahead Tips

Prepare the soup in advance and refrigerate for a fast reheatable dish.

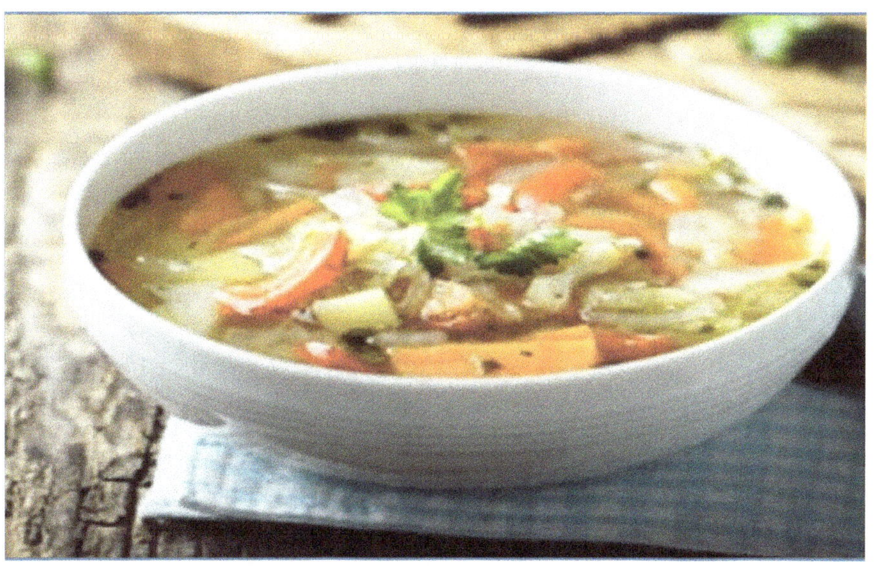

Ravioli & Vegetable Soup

Ravioli & Vegetable Soup is a medley of vibrant vegetables, tender ravioli, and aromatic herbs. This wholesome soup is a celebration of flavors in every spoonful.

Cooking/Prep Time: 25 mins | Servings: 2

Ingredients

- 1 tablespoon of olive oil
- One onion, diced
- Two carrots, sliced
- Two celery stalks, chopped
- 2 cloves of garlic, minced
- Four cups of vegetable broth
- A can (15 oz) of diced tomatoes
- 1 cup of fresh or frozen ravioli
- One zucchini, diced
- A teaspoon of Italian seasoning
- Salt and pepper to your desired preference
- Fresh basil for garnish

Directions

1. Pour olive oil into a big saucepan and bring it heat over medium flame. Pour in the garlic, onion, carrots, and celery. Allow it sauté until tender.
2. Add the chopped tomatoes and the veggie broth. Bring to a simmer.
3. Add the salt, pepper, zucchini, and Italian seasoning. Sauté the ravioli till they are soft.
4. Before serving, sprinkle some fresh basil on top.

Nutritional Value (Per Serving)

Calories: 320 | Carbs: 45g | Protein: 10g | Fats: 12g | Fiber: 8g

Tips

For a time-saving option, use frozen ravioli and keep them in the freezer until ready to cook.

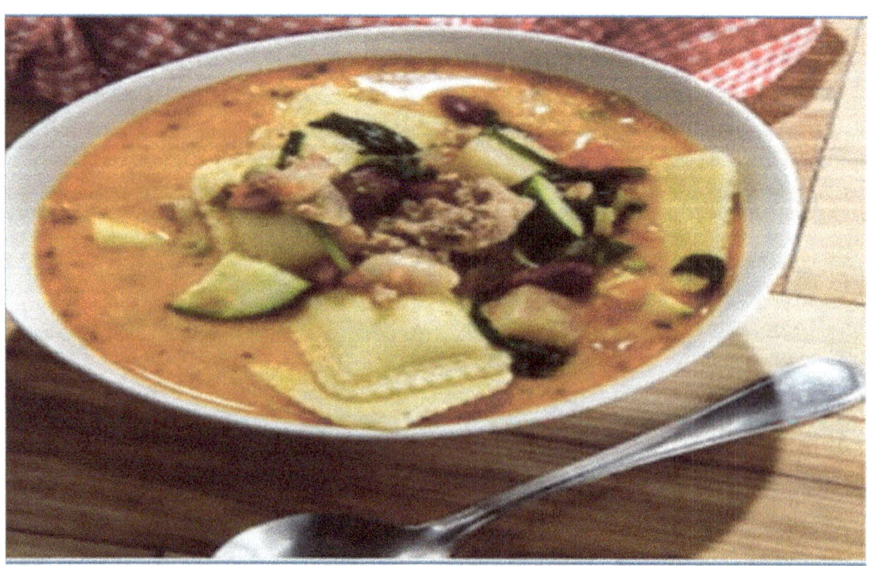

White Bean Soup with Tomato and Shrimp

Savor the delicate flavors of the Mediterranean with White Bean prepared with Tomato and Shrimp—a delightful combination of creamy white beans, juicy tomatoes, and succulent shrimp.

 Cooking/Prep Time: 25 mins Servings: 2

Ingredients

- One tablespoon of olive oil
- 1 onion, diced
- Two cloves of garlic, minced
- 15 oz / 1 can of white beans, rinsed and strained
- 1 can (15 oz) of diced tomatoes
- One cup of shrimp, peeled and deveined
- Four cups of chicken or vegetable broth
- A teaspoon of oregano
- Season to taste
- Fresh parsley for garnish

Directions

1. Heat up the olive oil in a saucepan over a low flame. Add the garlic and onion and sauté until tender.

2. Add the broth, oregano, shrimp, chopped tomatoes, white beans, salt, and pepper. Cook till the shrimp is tender.

3. Before serving, garnish with fresh parsley.

Nutritional Value (Per Serving)

Calories: 290 | Carbs: 30g | Protein: 20g | Fats: 10g | Fiber: 8g

Make Ahead Tips

For added depth, use fire-roasted diced tomatoes.

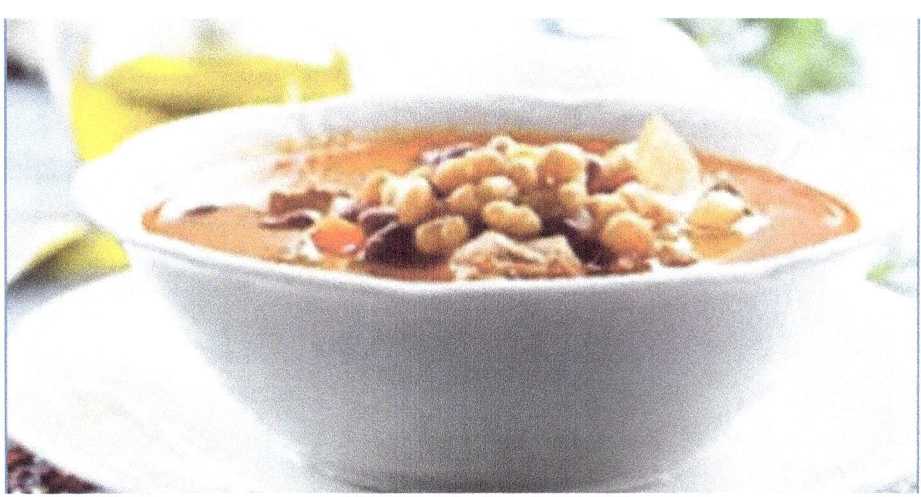

Chicken & White Bean Soup

This heartwarming soup is a testament to the wholesome simplicity of Mediterranean flavors.

 Cooking/Prep Time: 40 mins Servings: 2

Ingredients

- A tablespoon of olive oil
- 1 onion, diced
- Two carrots, sliced
- Two celery stalks, chopped
- 2 cloves of garlic, minced
- Eight oz of chicken breast, cooked and shredded
- A can (15 oz) of white beans, drained and rinsed
- 4 cups of chicken broth
- 1 teaspoon of rosemary
- Salt and pepper to preference
- Fresh parsley for garnish

Directions

1. Warm the olive oil in a saucepan over a medium flame. Add the garlic, onion, celery, and carrots. Cook until the veggies get tender.
2. Add the white beans, chicken stock, shredded chicken, salt, and pepper. Cook until well heated.
3. Before serving, sprinkle some fresh parsley on top.

Make Ahead Tips:

For a time-saving option, use pre-cooked rotisserie chicken.

Note:

Rotisserie chicken has high sodium, however, you might need to adjust the salt used.

Nutritional Value (Per Serving)

Calories: 320 | Carbs: 30g | Protein: 25g | Fats: 10g | Fiber: 8g

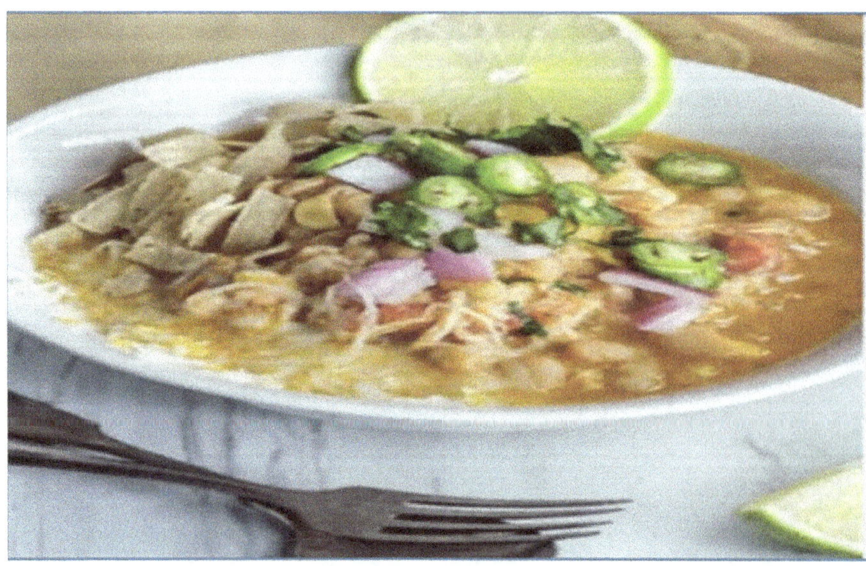

Vegan Cabbage Soup

This Vegan Cabbage Soup—is a hearty blend of vegetables, beans, and cabbage. It is not only flavorful but also an excellent source of plant-based nutrition.

 Cooking/Prep Time: 35 mins 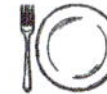 Servings: 2

Ingredients

- Two sausages, sliced
- One tablespoon of olive oil
- 1 onion, diced
- Two cloves of garlic, minced
- 2 cups of Brussels sprouts, halved
- Two potatoes, diced
- 4 cups of chicken or vegetable broth
- 1 teaspoon of thyme
- Season to taste
- Parmesan cheese for garnish

Nutritional Value (Per Serving)

Calories: 380 | Carbs: 30g | Protein: 18g | Fats: 22g | Fiber: 8g

Directions

1. Saute sausage pieces in a saucepan until they are browned. Take out and put aside.
2. Pour olive oil into the same saucepan and allow to heat under medium flame. Add the Brussels sprouts, onion, and garlic. Sauté the veggies till they get soft.
3. Add the broth, potatoes, salt, pepper, and thyme. Cook until the potatoes are tender.
4. Return the cooked sausage to the pot.
5. Garnish with Parmesan cheese and serve.

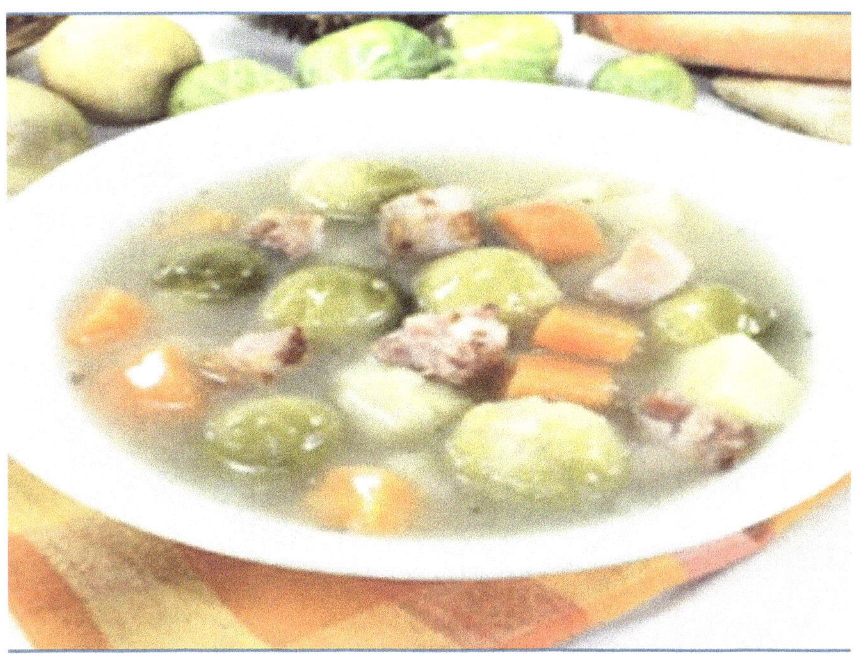

Slow-Cooker Mediterranean Diet Stew

This Vegan Cabbage Soup—is a hearty blend of vegetables, beans, and cabbage. It is not only flavorful but also an excellent source of plant-based nutrition.

 Cooking/Prep Time: 6hrs 45 mins   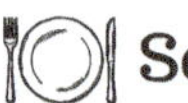 Servings: 2

Ingredients

- 1 can of no-salt-added fire-roasted diced tomatoes
- One and a half cups of low-sodium vegetable broth
- Half a cup of coarsely chopped onion
- ¾ cup chopped carrot
- 1 clove of garlic, minced
- A quarter teaspoon of dried oregano
- ¾ teaspoon of salt
- ¾ quarter teaspoon of crushed red pepper
- ¾ teaspoon of ground pepper
- 1 can of no-salt-added chickpeas, rinsed, divided
- A bunch of lacinato kale stemmed and chopped (about 8 cups)
- ½ tablespoon of lemon juice
- 2 tablespoons extra-virgin olive oil
- Fresh basil leaves, torn if large
- 2 lemon wedges (Optional)

Nutritional Value (Per Serving)

Calories: 191 | Carbs: 23g | Protein: 6g | Fats: 8g | Fiber: 10g

Directions

1. In a 4-quart slow cooker, combine tomatoes, broth, onion, carrot, garlic, oregano, salt, crushed red pepper, and pepper. Cook on Low for six hours with a cover on.

2. Pour 1/4 cup of the slow cooker's cooking liquid into a small basin. Add the two tablespoons of chickpeas and mash them well with a fork.

3. To the mixture in the slow cooker, add the mashed chickpeas, greens, lemon juice, and the remaining whole chickpeas. Mix everything together. After the kale is soft, approximately 30 minutes, simmer it covered on Low.

4. Evenly divide the stew between two dishes and pour in some oil. Add basil as a garnish. If preferred, enjoy with slices of lemon.

Make Ahead Tips

For added richness, stir in a dollop of pesto before serving.

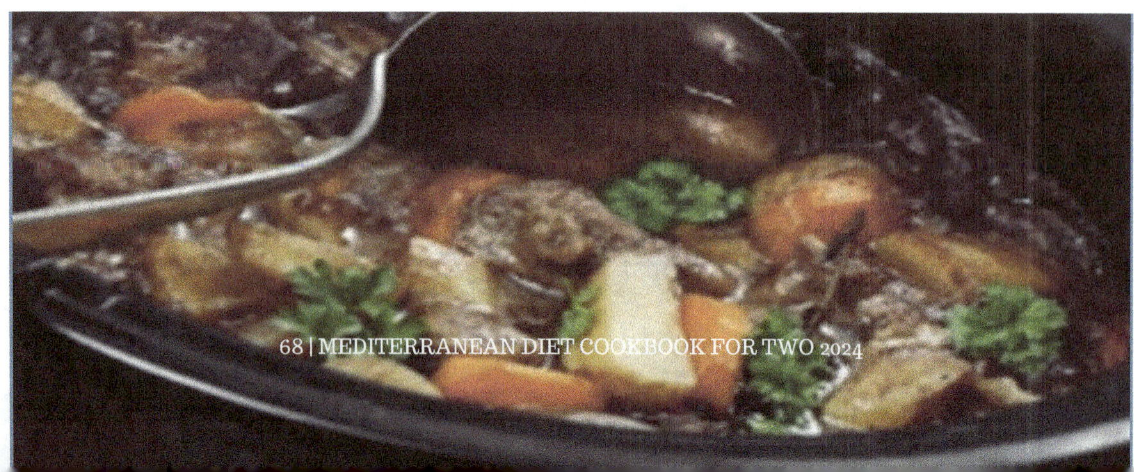

Slow-Cooker Mediterranean Diet Stew

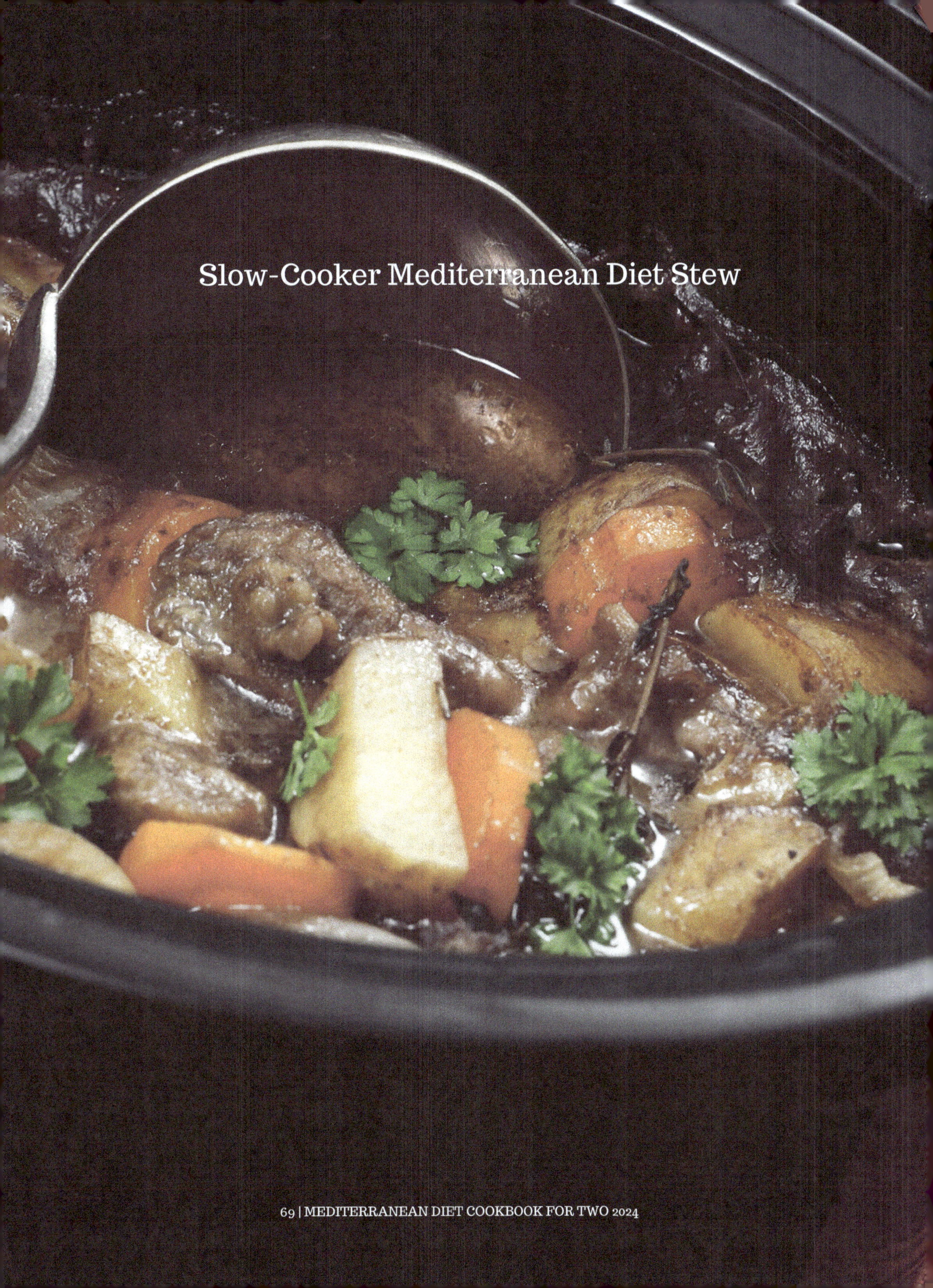

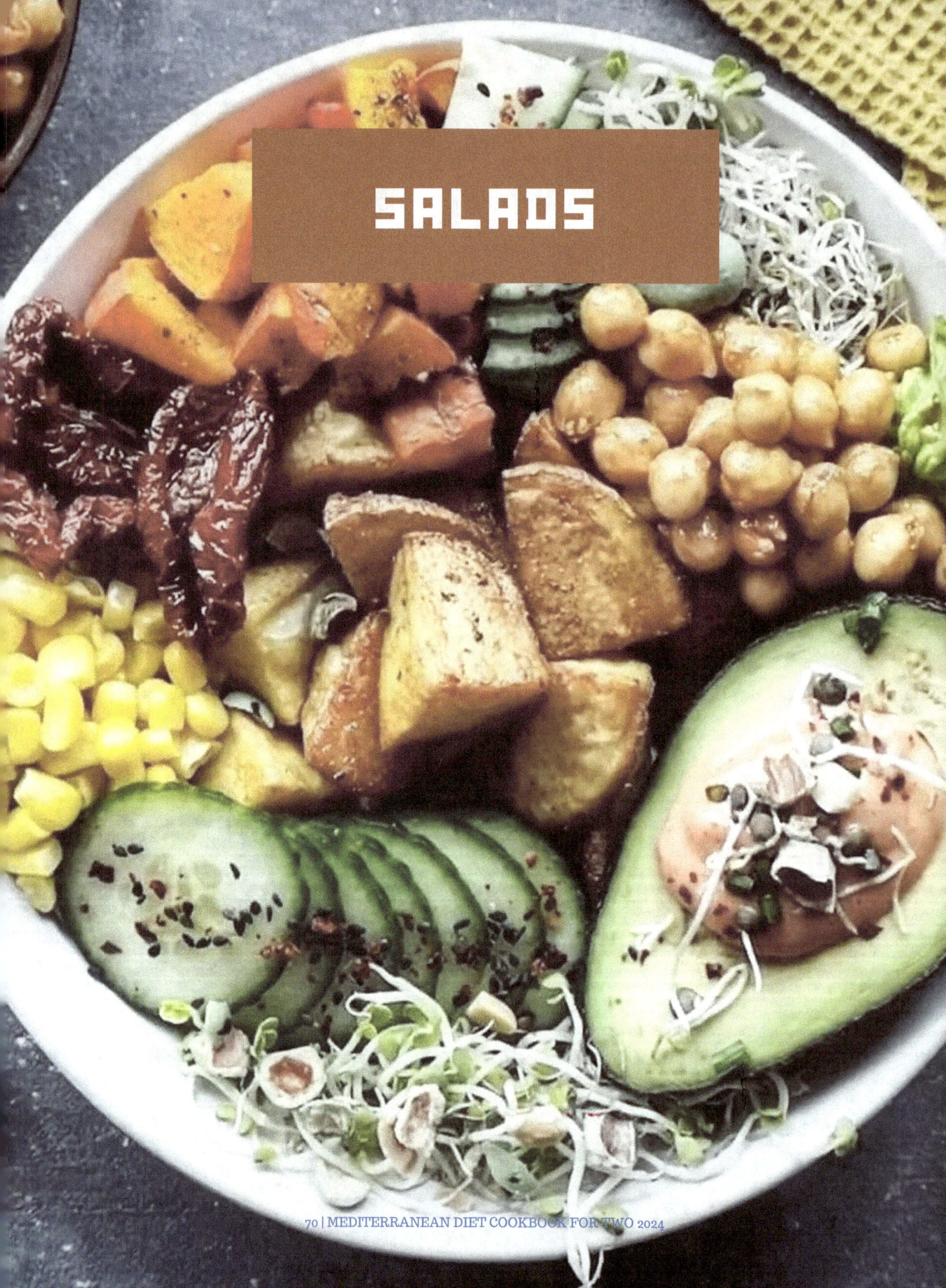
SALADS

Kale, Quinoa & Apple Salad

This vibrant salad is a blend of flavors and textures that will leave you feeling satisfied and nourished.

 Cooking/Prep Time: 20 mins   Servings: 2

Ingredients

- One tablespoon of cider vinegar
- Half a tablespoon of pure maple syrup
- 1/4 teaspoon of salt
- 1/8 teaspoon of ground pepper
- 1/8 cup of extra-virgin olive oil
- 1 medium bunch curly kale, stemmed, thinly chopped (like 4 cups)
- One medium Honeycrisp apple, unpeeled, roughly chopped
- 1 small fennel bulb, cored and thinly sliced (1 and 1/2 cups)
- 1 cup of cooked quinoa, chilled or normal temp.
- 1/4 cup of slivered almonds, toasted
- 1/6 cup of dried cherries
- 1/4 cup crumbled blue cheese

Directions

1. In a large bowl, whisk together vinegar, maple syrup, salt, and pepper. Drizzle in the oil gradually while stirring to blend.

2. With clean hands, add the kale and massage it into the dressing for three to five minutes, or until it's fully coated and somewhat soft.

3. Toss to blend the quinoa, apples, and fennel. Distribute over 2 dishes and garnish with blue cheese, cherries, and almonds.

Tips

- Before using nuts in a dish, toast them for the finest taste. To toast the nuts, set them in a small dry pan over medium-low heat and stir regularly for 2 to 4 minutes, or until aromatic.
- For a soft texture, rub some olive oil into the kale before assembling the salad

Nutritional Value (Per Serving)

Calories: 350 | Carbs: 35g | Protein: 10g | Fats: 20g | Fiber: 6g

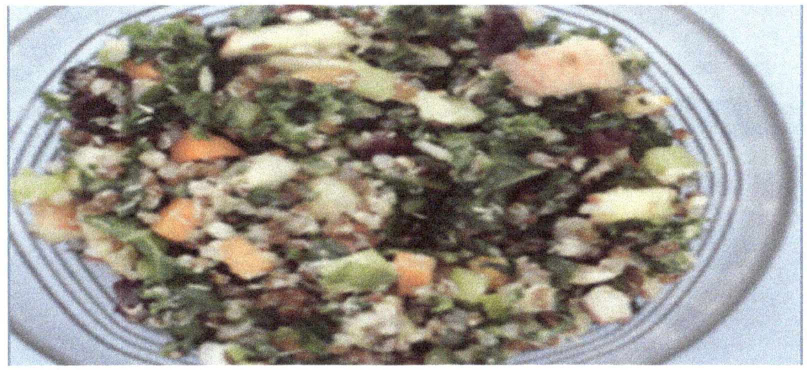

Avocado Tuna Salad

Enjoy this Avocado Tuna Salad—a delightful blend of creamy avocado, protein-packed tuna, and vibrant veggies.

 Cooking/Prep Time: 15 mins   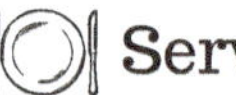 Servings: 2

Ingredients

- 1 can (5 oz) tuna, drained
- 1 avocado, diced
- 1 cup cherry tomatoes, halved
- 1/4 cup red onion, finely chopped
- 2 tablespoons fresh parsley, chopped
- 1 tablespoon olive oil
- 1 tablespoon lemon juice
- ¼ teaspoon of salt
- ⅛ teaspoon of ground pepper to taste

Directions

1. Mix the chopped avocado, cherry tomatoes, red onion, fresh parsley, and drained tuna in a bowl.
2. Pour lemon juice and olive oil over the salad. Stir gently.
3. Add pepper and salt according to taste or as in the ingredients.

Tips

- For a refreshing twist, add a splash of balsamic vinegar to the dressing.

Nutritional Value (Per Serving)

Calories: 280 | Carbs: 15g | Protein: 20g | Fats: 18g | Fiber: 6g

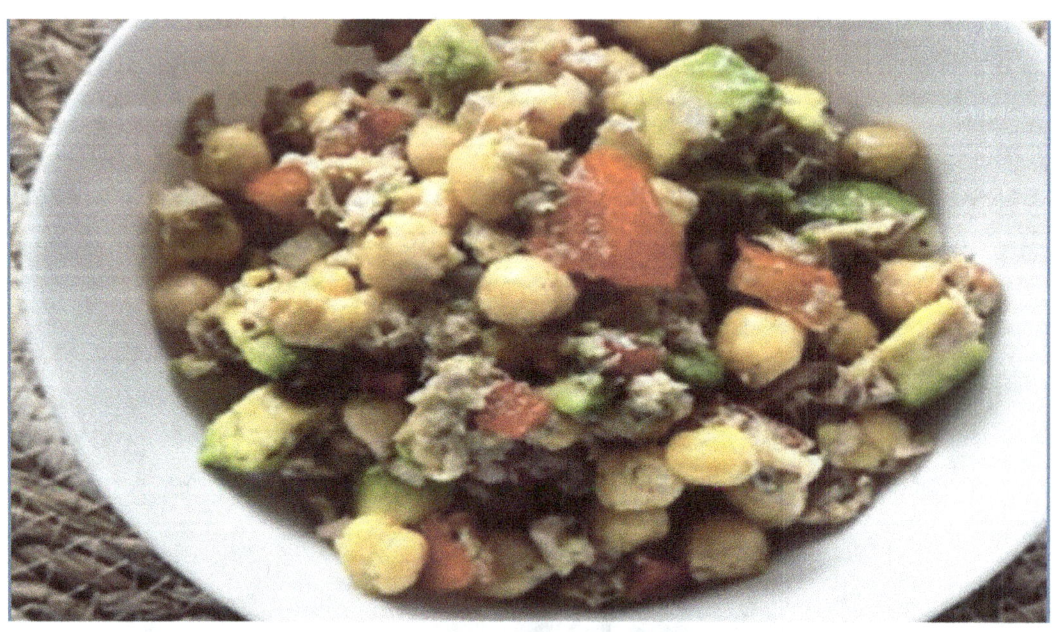

Lemony Lentil Salad with Feta

This Mediterranean-inspired salad is a nutritious and flavorful addition to your meal.

 Cooking/Prep Time: 25 mins 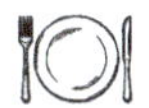 Servings: 2

Ingredients

- One cup of cooked green lentils
- 1/4 cup of feta cheese, crumbled
- 1/2 a cucumber, diced
- A quarter teaspoon of salt
- Ground pepper, ⅛ teaspoon
- 1/4 cup of red bell pepper, diced
- Two tablespoons of red onion, finely chopped
- 2 tablespoons of fresh mint, chopped
- Two tablespoons of olive oil
- Half a tablespoon of lemon zest
- 2 tablespoons lemon juice

Directions

1. Place the cooked lentils, chopped cucumber, red bell pepper, red onion, feta cheese, salt, pepper, and fresh mint in a bowl.
2. Whisk the olive oil, lemon zest, and lemon juice in a separate small bowl.
3. After adding the dressing, carefully mix the salad until it is thoroughly covered.

Tips:

Allow the salad to chill in the refrigerator for an hour before serving for enhanced flavors.

Nutritional Value (Per Serving)

Calories: 320 | Carbs: 30g | Protein: 15g | Fats: 15g | Fiber: 12g

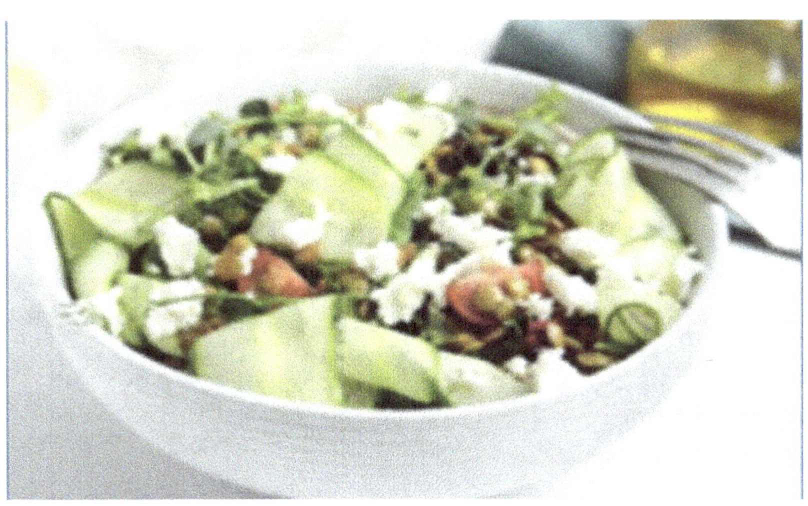

Salad Primavera with Creamy Mustard Vinaigrette

This salad is not only visually appealing but also a nourishing feast for your taste buds.

 Cooking/Prep Time: 20 mins 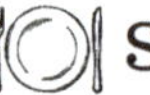 Servings: 2

Ingredients

- 4 cups of mixed salad greens
- A cup of cherry tomatoes, halved
- 1/2 cup of cucumber, sliced
- Half a cup of carrots, julienned
- 1/4 cup of radishes, thinly sliced
- Two tablespoons of pine nuts
- 2 tablespoons of olive oil
- 1 tablespoon Dijon mustard
- Salt, ¼ teaspoon
- 1 tablespoon balsamic vinegar
- 1 tablespoon Greek yogurt
- Ground pepper, about ⅛ teaspoon

Nutritional Value (Per Serving)

Calories: 280 | Carbs: 18g | Protein: 7g | Fats: 22g | Fiber: 6g

Directions

1. Combine mixed salad greens, cucumber, cherry tomatoes, carrots, radishes, and pine nuts in a big bowl.
2. To make the creamy mustard vinaigrette, combine olive oil, Dijon mustard, balsamic vinegar, Greek yogurt, salt, and pepper in a small bowl.
3. Pour the vinaigrette over the salad and gently toss until well-coated.

Tips

- To maintain crispiness, keep the dressing separate until ready to serve.

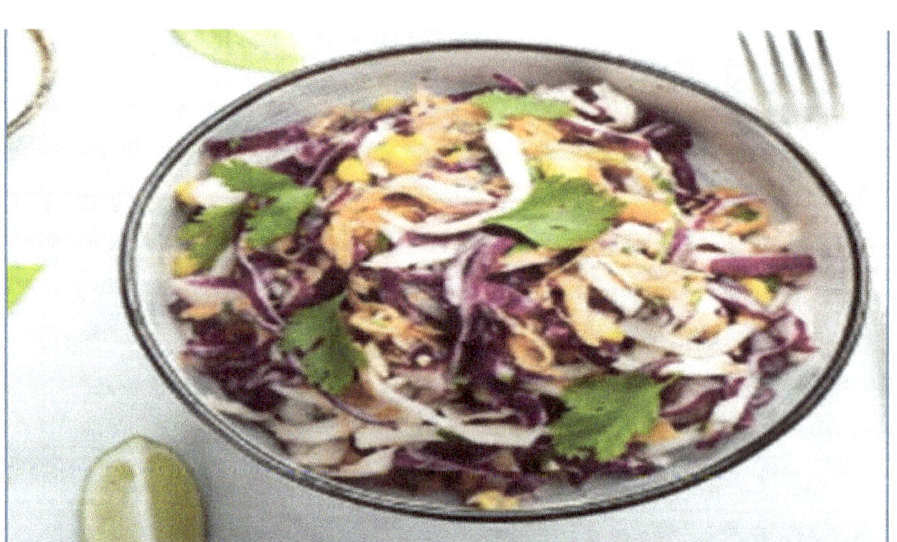

Purple Fruit Salad

This colorful salad is not only visually appealing but also a nutritious way to satisfy your sweet cravings.

 Cooking/Prep Time: 15 mins 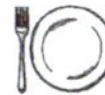 Servings: 2

Ingredients

- One cup of purple grapes, halved
- 1 cup of blackberries
- A cup of blueberries
- 1/2 cup of pomegranate seeds
- Two tablespoons of fresh mint, chopped
- 1 tablespoon honey
- A tablespoon of lime juice

Nutritional Value (Per Serving)

Calories: 180 | Carbs: 45g | Protein: 2g | Fats: 1g | Fiber: 8g

Directions

1. Gather the blueberries, pomegranate seeds, purple grapes, blackberries, and fresh mint in a container.
2. Mix the honey and lime juice in a small basin.
3. Splash with the honey-lime dressing and toss gently till evenly coated.

Make Ahead/Cooking Tips

- Prepare the dressing separately and add it just before serving to maintain the freshness of the fruits.

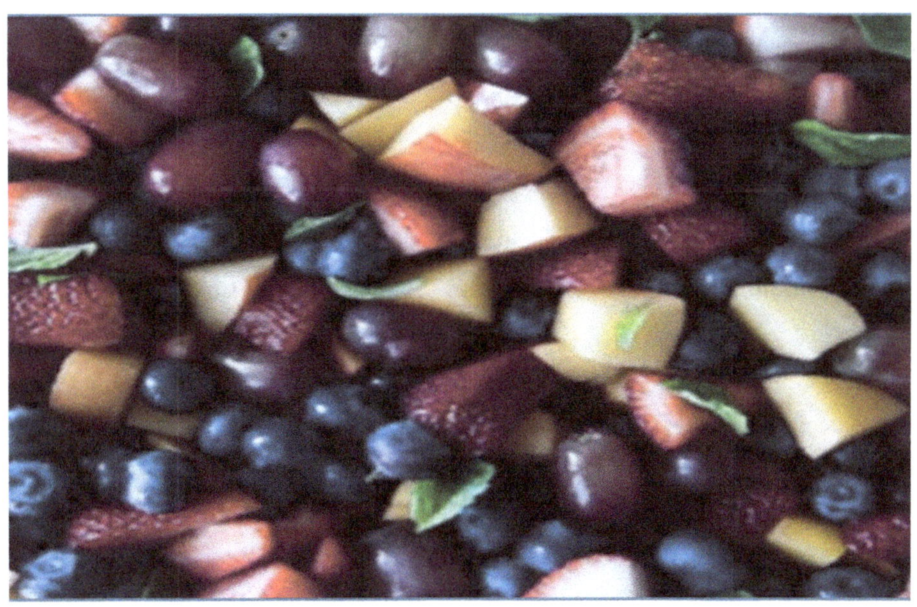

Falafel Salad with Lemon-Tahini Dressing

Enjoy this hearty Falafel Salad with Lemon-Tahini Dressing—a harmonious blend of crispy falafel, fresh veggies, and a zesty tahini dressing.

 Cooking/Prep Time: 30 mins  Servings: 2

Ingredients

- Four falafel patties, cooked and crumbled
- 4 cups of mixed salad greens
- One cucumber, diced
- 1 tomato, diced
- 1/8 ground pepper
- 1/4 cup of red onion, thinly sliced
- A quarter cup of Kalamata olives, pitted and halved
- 1/4 cup of feta cheese, crumbled
- Two tablespoons of tahini
- 2 tablespoons water
- One tablespoon of lemon juice
- 1 clove of garlic, minced
- Salt (quarter teaspoon)

Directions

1. Combine mixed salad greens, diced cucumber, diced tomato, chopped red onion, crumbled falafel, and Kalamata olives in a big bowl.
2. To make the lemon-tahini dressing, combine tahini, water, lemon juice, chopped garlic, salt, and pepper in a small bowl.
3. Over the salad, drizzle with the dressing and mix gently until completely incorporated.

Nutritional Value (Per Serving)

Calories: 420 | Carbs: 35g | Protein: 14g | Fats: 26g | Fiber: 10g

Tips

- Reheat falafel patties briefly before serving for a warm contrast to the crisp salad.

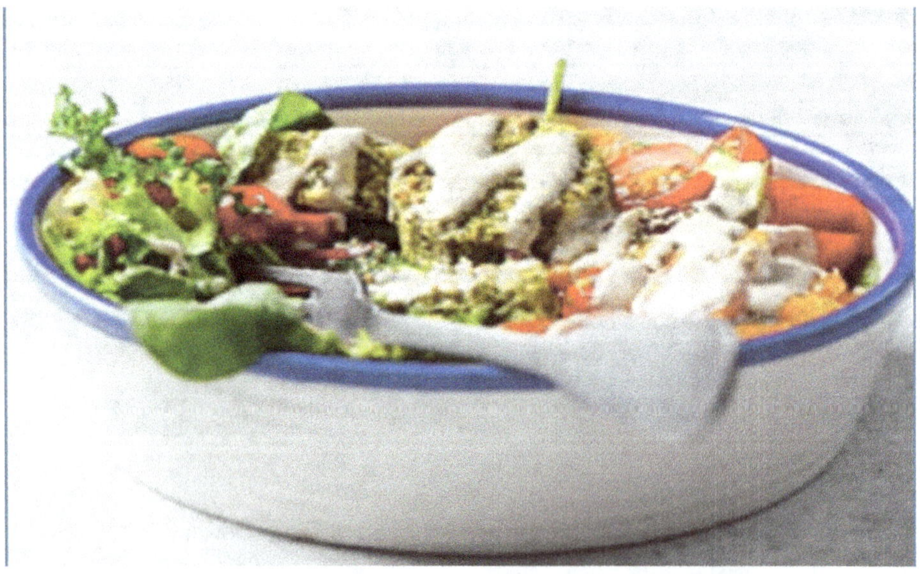

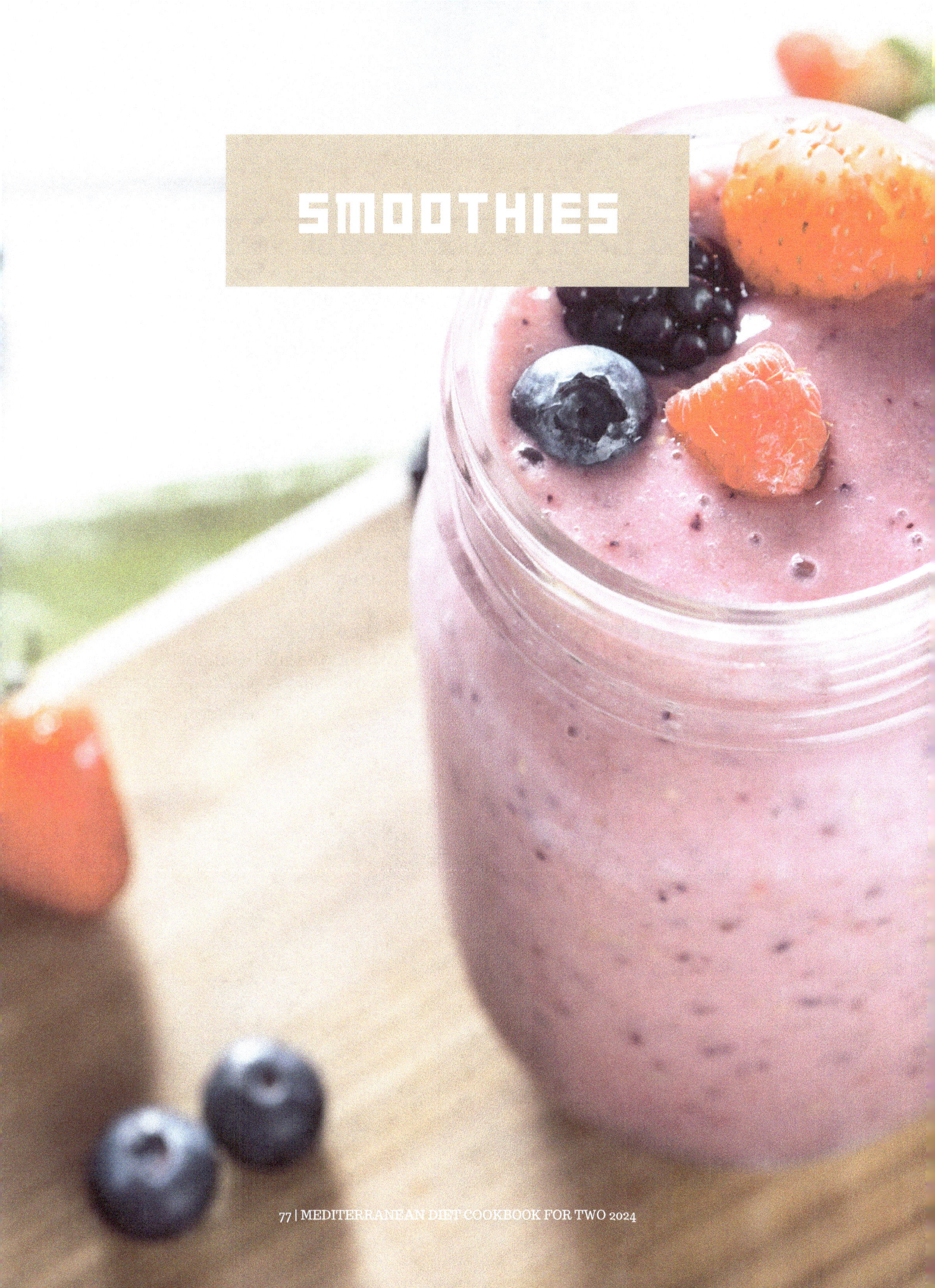

SMOOTHIES

SMOOTHIES

Strawberry-Banana Green Smoothie

This smoothie is a refreshing and wholesome way to fuel your morning.

 Cooking/Prep Time: 10 mins | Servings: 2

Ingredients

- A cup of fresh strawberries, hulled
- 1 ripe banana
- One cup of fresh spinach leaves
- 1/2 a cup of Greek yogurt
- Half a cup of almond milk
- 1 tablespoon of chia seeds
- Ice cubes (optional)

Nutritional Value (Per Serving)

Calories: 180 | Carbs: 25g | Protein: 8g | Fats: 6g | Fiber: 7g

Directions

1. Put together fresh spinach leaves, ripe banana, strawberries, Greek yogurt, almond milk, and chia seeds in a blender.
2. Blend till creamy and smooth.
3. If you want a more refreshing consistency, add ice cubes.

Make Ahead Tips

- Prep individual smoothie packs with pre-measured ingredients for a quick and efficient morning routine.

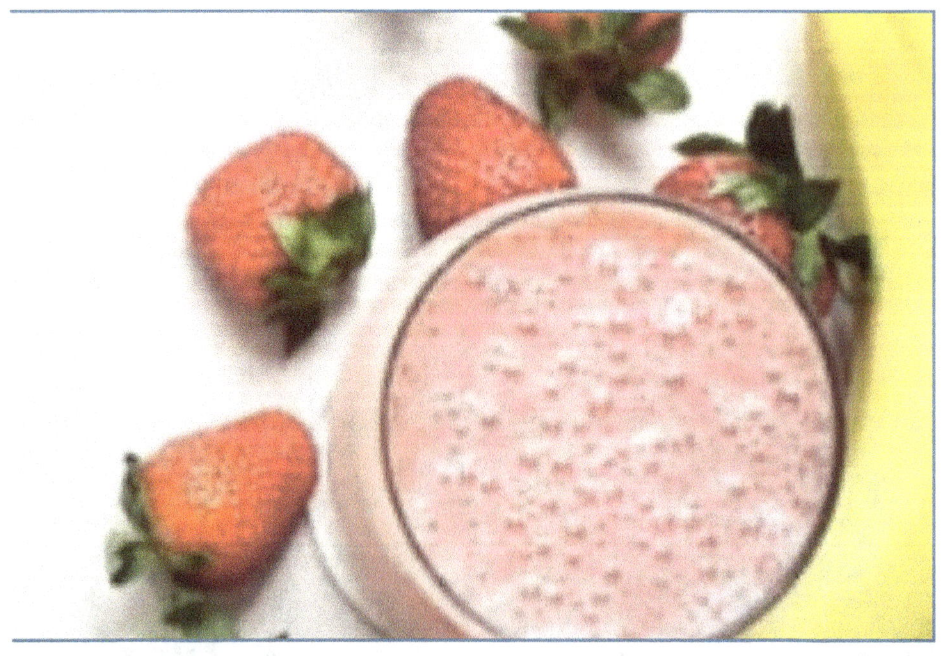

Fruit & Yogurt Smoothie

This smoothie is not only delicious but also a source of essential nutrients to power up your day.

 Cooking/Prep Time: 15 mins Servings: 2

Ingredients

- A cup of mixed berries (blueberries/strawberries/raspberries)
- 1/2 a cup mango chunks
- Half cup of pineapple chunks
- 1/2 a cup Greek yogurt
- Half cup of orange juice
- 1 tablespoon of honey
- Ice cubes (if preferred)

Directions

1. Blend together mixed berries, Greek yogurt, orange juice, honey, and pieces of mango and pineapple in a blender.
2. Pulse till creamy and smooth.
3. To get a cold texture, feel free to add ice cubes.

Nutritional Value (Per Serving)

Calories: 220 | Carbs: 40g | Protein: 9g | Fats: 4g | Fiber: 6g

Tips

- Freeze fruits in advance for a thicker and frosty consistency

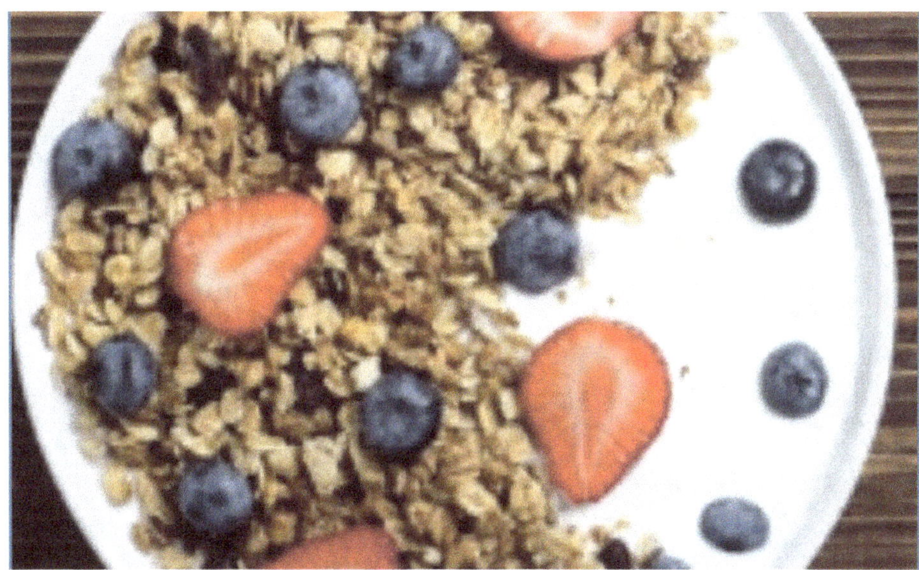

Kale & Apple Smoothie

This nutrient-packed smoothie is a delightful blend of freshness and health.

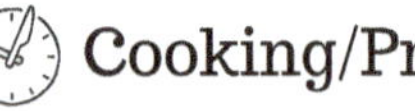 Cooking/Prep Time: 12 mins   Servings: 2

Ingredients

- 2 cups of kale leaves, stems removed
- One apple, cored and chopped
- Half a banana
- 1/2 cup of plain Greek yogurt
- Half a cup of orange juice
- 1 tablespoon of flax seeds
- Ice cubes (as desired)

Directions

1. Blend together the diced apple, banana, Greek yogurt, orange juice, and flax seeds with the kale leaves.
2. Combine till clear and creamy.
3. If you would want something more chilly, add some ice cubes.

Nutritional Value (Per Serving)

Calories: 200 | Carbs: 35g | Protein:10g | Fats: 5g | Fiber: 8g

Make Ahead Tips

- Pre-cut and freeze kale for an easy-to-use, prepped ingredient.

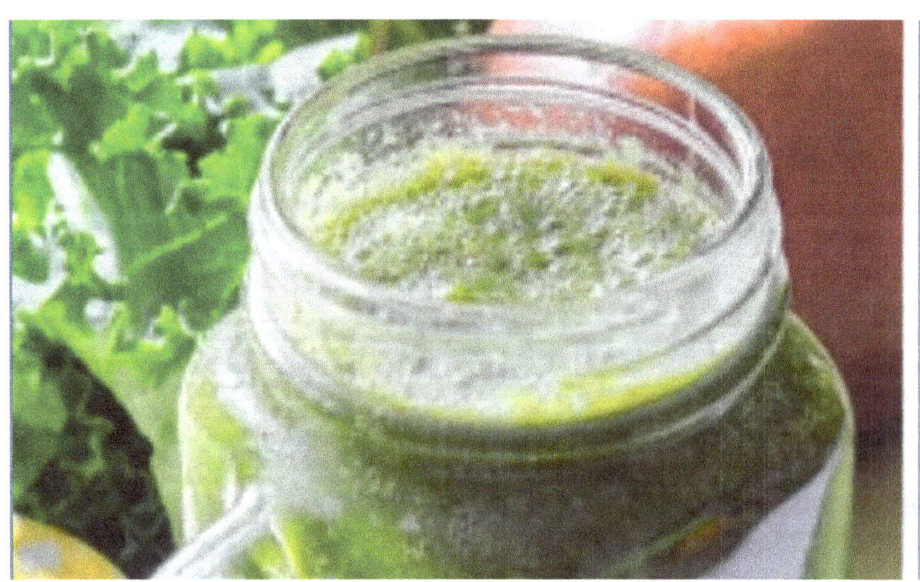

Mixed-Berry Breakfast Smoothie

This smoothie is a delightful way to incorporate antioxidant-rich berries into your morning routine that's both satisfying and nutritious.

 Cooking/Prep Time: 10 mins 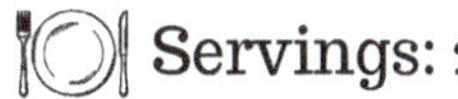 Servings: 2

Ingredients

- A cup of mixed berries (blackberries/strawberries/blueberries)
- 1/2 cup of plain Greek yogurt
- Half a cup of rolled oats
- One tablespoon of almond butter
- 1 tablespoon of honey
- ½ a cup almond milk
- Ice

Nutritional Value (Per Serving)

Calories: 250 | Carbs: 40g | Protein:12g | Fats: 7g | Fiber: 8g

Directions

1. Blend mixed berries, rolled oats, Greek yogurt, almond butter, honey, and almond milk in a blender.
2. Beat till creamy and smooth.
3. Add ice cubes for a refreshing chill.

Tips

- To get a more smooth texture, soak oats in almond milk.

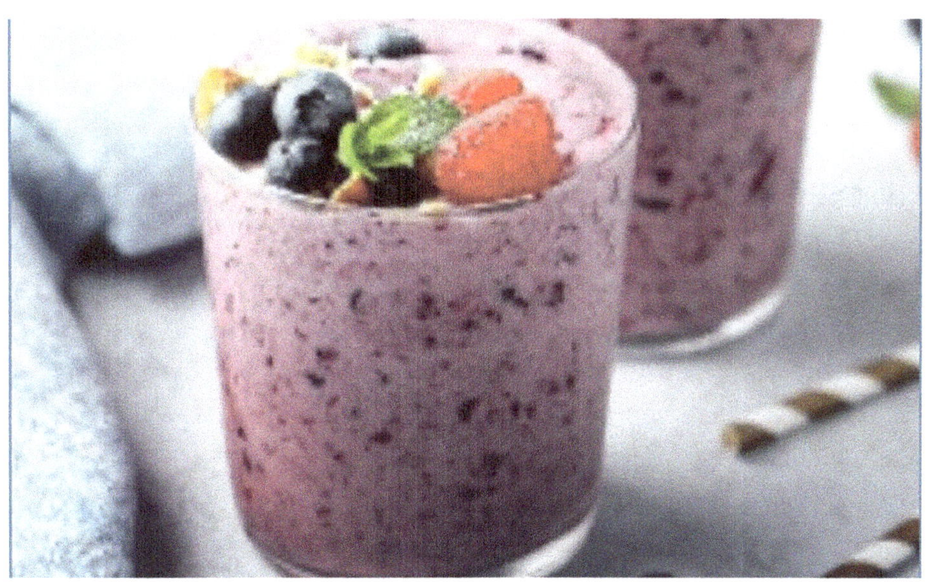

Vegan Smoothie Bowl

This smoothie bowl is not just a feast for the eyes but a wholesome start to your day.

 Cooking/Prep Time: 15 mins   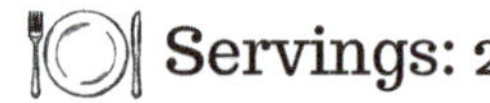 Servings: 2

Ingredients

- 2 frozen bananas
- One cup of frozen mixed berries
- 1/2 a cup almond milk
- One tablespoon of chia seeds

Toppings: shredded coconut, sliced kiwi, granola, and pumpkin seeds

Nutritional Value (Per Serving)

Calories: 280 | Carbs: 55g | Protein:5g | Fats: 7g | Fiber: 12g

Directions

1. Beat frozen mixed berries, frozen bananas, and almond milk in a blender until smooth.
2. Transfer the smoothie mixture to bowls.
3 Add pumpkin seeds, granola, shredded coconut, and sliced kiwi on top.

Make Ahead Tips

- Pre-slice and freeze bananas and berries for a thicker consistency.

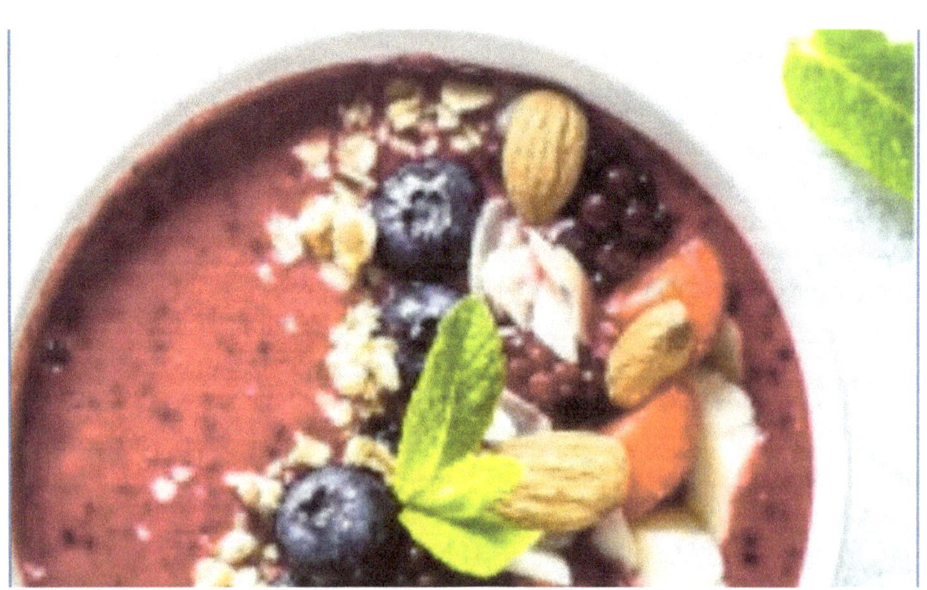

Raspberry-Kefir Power Smoothie

This smoothie is a powerhouse of probiotics, antioxidants, and essential nutrients.

 Cooking/Prep Time: 12 mins   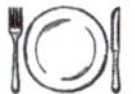 Servings: 2

Ingredients

- One cup of fresh raspberries
- 1 cup of kefir
- ½ a banana
- A tablespoon of hemp seeds
- 1 tablespoon of pumpkin seeds
- One tablespoon of honey
- Ice cubes (optional)

Directions

1. Fresh raspberries, kefir, banana, hemp seeds, pumpkin seeds, and honey should all be combined in a blender.
2. Blend until creamy and silky smooth.
3. For a chilly texture, feel free to add ice cubes.

Nutritional Value (Per Serving)

Calories: 230 | Carbs: 30g | Protein:9g | Fats: 8g | Fiber: 7g

Tips

- Include a scoop of protein powder for an added energy boost.

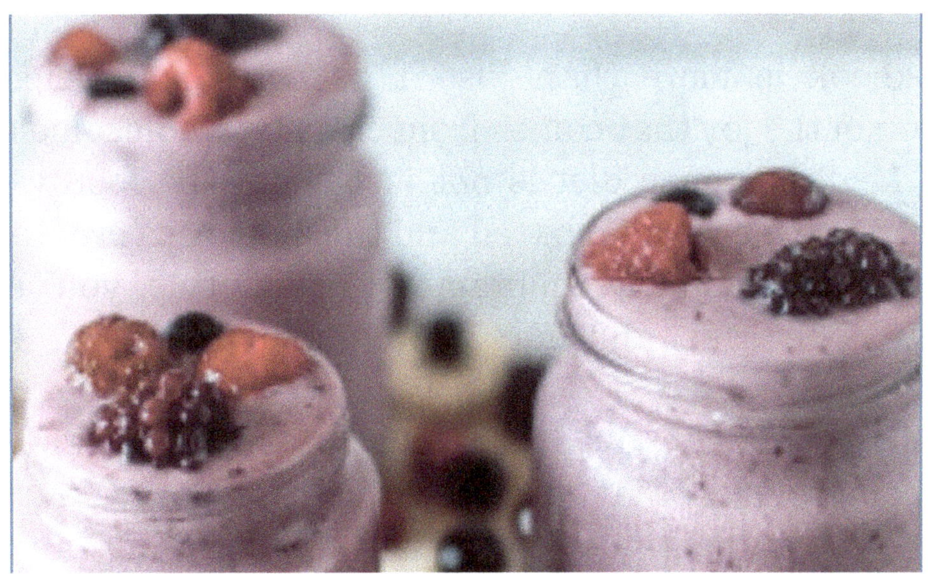

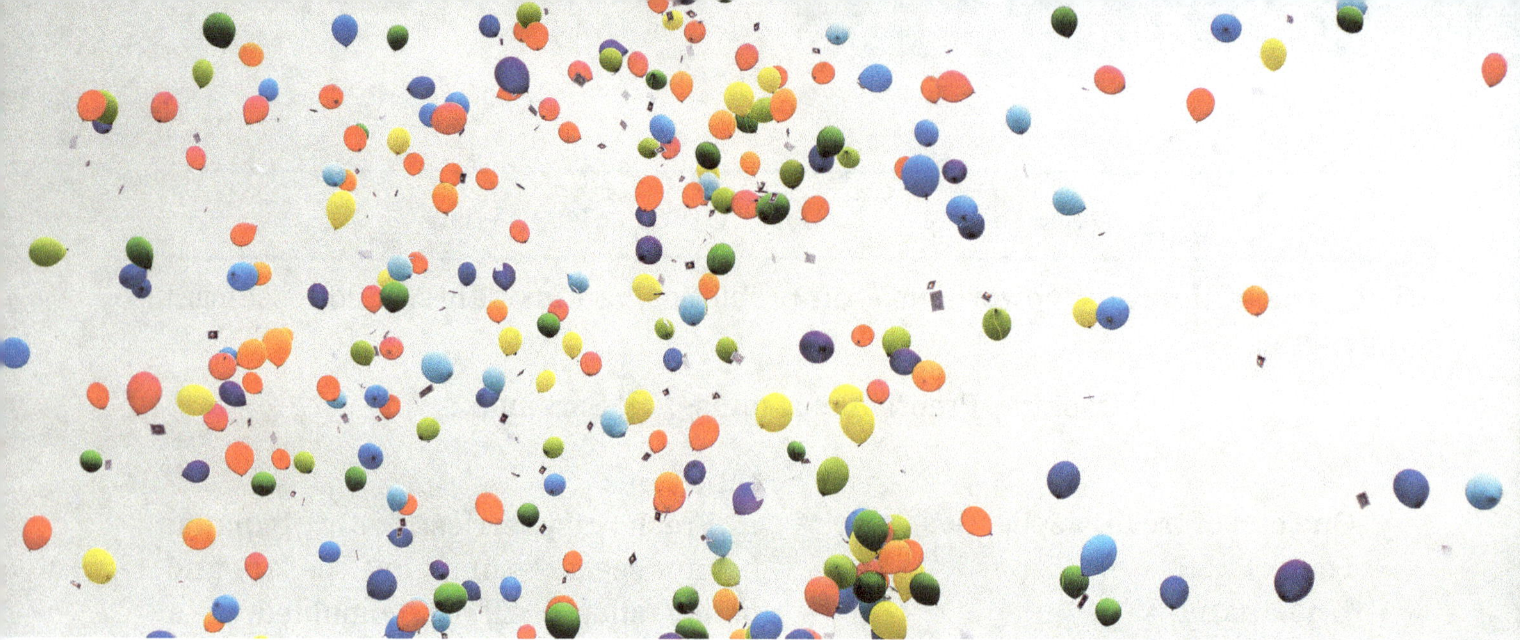

CONCLUSION

Congratulations on reaching the final pages of "Mediterranean Diet Cookbook For Two," I hope this culinary journey has been as ecstatic for you as it has been for me. Nourishing your body and tantalizing your taste buds is a journey, and I'm honored to have been your guide through the vibrant and health-conscious world of Mediterranean cuisine.

This cookbook is more than just a collection of recipes; it's a celebration of the joy that comes from crafting wholesome meals for two. The Mediterranean diet is not just about the food we eat but also about the experiences shared and the memories created around the table. I believe that by embracing this lifestyle, you've taken a step toward a healthier and more joyful way of living.

Your kitchen is now a canvas, and you, the artist, have the power to create masterpieces that are both delicious and nurturing. I encourage you to continue experimenting, adapting, and making these recipes your own. Let the spirit of the Mediterranean infuse your daily life, transforming the way you approach food and well-being.

Thank you for allowing this guide to be a part of your culinary adventure. Your support means the world to me, and I'm genuinely grateful for the trust you've placed in these recipes.

If you have any questions, want to share your experiences, or find yourself in need of guidance, please feel free to reach out to me at therealjessiejclarke@gmail.com.

Your opinions, observations, and any inventive modifications you've made to the recipes would be much appreciated. Your suggestions are very helpful and will surely influence future releases. It's also a great opportunity to spread the love and teach others about the delights of preparing Mediterranean food for two.

I'm wishing you health and many happy cooking moments!

Warmest regards!

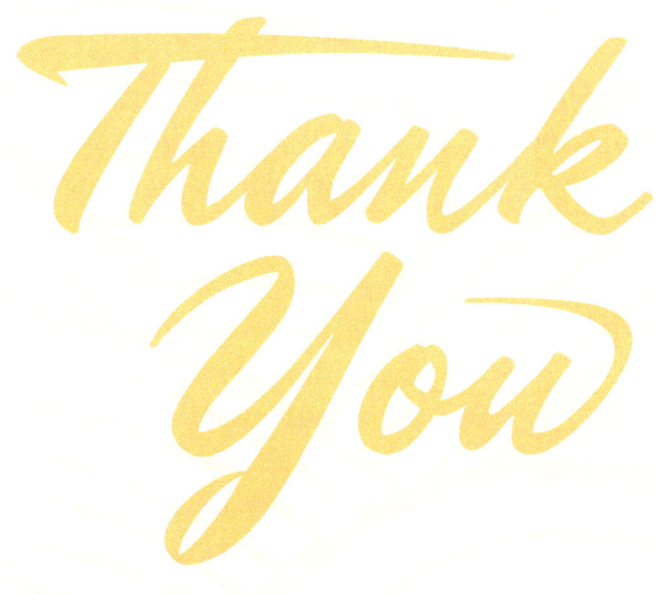

MEASUREMENTS AND CONVERSIONS TABLE

Use the below handy table to ensure precision and success in your culinary endeavors. Happy cooking!

VOLUME MEASUREMENTS:

1 teaspoon (tsp) = 5 milliliters (ml)

1 tablespoon (tbsp) = 15 milliliters (ml)

1 fluid ounce (fl oz) = 30 milliliters (ml)

1 cup = 240 milliliters (ml)

1 pint (2 cups) = 480 milliliters (ml)

1 quart (4 cups) = 960 milliliters (ml)

1 gallon (16 cups) = 3,840 milliliters (ml)

WEIGHT MEASUREMENTS:

1 ounce (oz) = 28 grams (g)

1 lb (pound) = 16 oz (ounces) = 454 g

DRY MEASUREMENTS:

1 cup (c) of flour or sugar = 120 grams (g)

1 cup (c) of nuts or chocolate chips = 150 grams (g)

BUTTER CONVERSIONS

1 stick of butter = 8 tablespoons = 1/2 cup = 113 grams (g)

LIQUID CONVERSIONS

A cup = 8 fluid oz = 240 ml

1 tablespoon = 1/2 fluid ounce = 15 milliliters (ml)

GRAINS AND LEGUMES:

1 cup of quinoa (uncooked) = 3 cups cooked

1 cup of lentils (uncooked) = 2.5 cups cooked

TEMPERATURE CONVERSIONS:

Fahrenheit to Celsius: (°F - 32) × 5/9 = °C

Celsius to Fahrenheit: (°C × 9/5) + 32 = °F

Oven Temperatures:

350°F = 180°C = Gas Mark 4

375°F = 190°C = Gas Mark 5

400°F = 200°C = Gas Mark 6

425°F = 220°C = Gas Mark 7

450°F = 230°C = Gas Mark 8

COMMON INGREDIENT EQUIVALENTS:

1 lemon yields approximately 2 tablespoons of juice

1 medium-sized onion is approximately 1 cup when chopped

1 clove of garlic is approximately 1 teaspoon when minced

1 medium-sized tomato is approximately 1 cup when diced

SWEETENERS:

1 cup of sugar = 200 grams (g)

1 cup of honey or maple syrup = 240 grams (g)

MISCELLANEOUS:

1 teaspoon of baking powder = 1/4 teaspoon of baking soda + 1/2 teaspoon of cream of tartar

1 cup of buttermilk = 1 cup of milk + 1 tablespoon of white vinegar or lemon juice (let sit for 5 minutes)

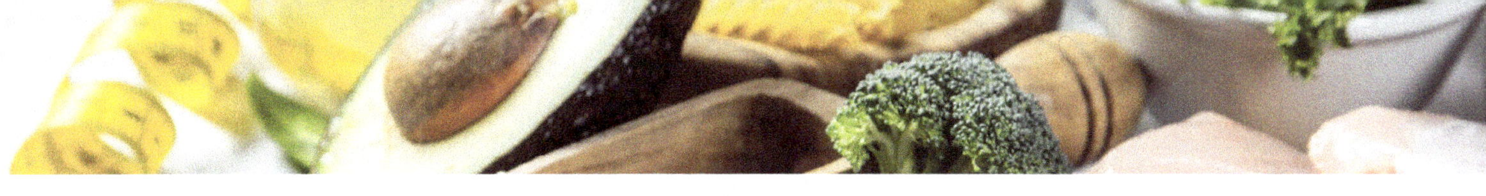

RECIPES INDEX